Changing Services for People with Learning Disabilities

Changing Services for People with Learning Disabilities

R. Farmer
Professor of Public Health Medicine

J. Rohde
Register Organizer

and

B. Sacks
Professor of Developmental Psychiatry

Charing Cross and Westminster Medical School, London, UK

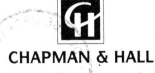

CHAPMAN & HALL

London · Glasgow · New York · Tokyo · Melbourne · Madras

Published by Chapman & Hall, 2–6 Boundary Row, London SE1 8HN

Chapman & Hall, 2–6 Boundary Row, London SE1 8HN, UK

Blackie Academic & Professional, Wester Cleddens Road, Bishopbriggs, Glasgow G64 2NZ, UK

Chapman & Hall, 29 West 35th Street, New York NY10001, USA

Chapman & Hall Japan, Thomson Publishing Japan, Hirakawacho Nemoto Building, 6F, 1–7–11 Hirakawa-cho, Chiyoda-ku, Tokyo 102, Japan

Chapman & Hall Australia, Thomas Nelson Australia, 102 Dodds Street, South Melbourne, Victoria 3205, Australia

Chapman & Hall India, R. Seshadri, 32 Second Main Road, CIT East, Madras 600 035, India

Distributed in the USA and Canada by Singular Publishing Group Inc., 4284 41st Street, San Diego, California 92105

First edition 1993

© 1993 R. Farmer, J. Rohde and B. Sacks

Typeset in 10/12 Palatino by Mews Photosetting, Beckenham, Kent
Printed in Great Britain by St Edmundsbury Press Ltd, Bury St Edmunds, Suffolk

ISBN 0 412 47480 8   1 56593 059 2 (USA)

A catalogue record for this book is available from the British Library

Library of Congress Cataloging-in-Publication data available

To people with mental handicaps
and their families in the hope of
a better future.

Contents

Contents

Acknowledgements

The assembling of so much detailed data about people with mental handicaps would not have been possible had it not been for the farsighted decisions of Dr Carl Burns, when he was the Area Medical Officer for the Kensington and Chelsea and Westminster Area Health Authority in the late 1970s, to sponsor the development of a Register rather than conduct occasional censuses. At a later stage, when the system had been established in Kensington and Chelsea and Westminster, Dr Jean Weddell, then at the North West Thames Regional Health Authority, made the decision to encourage the establishment of Registers in all the Districts in the Region.

Throughout the history of the development and maintenance of Registers in the Region a large number of people have given their commitment to the scheme. This work would not have been possible without the dedication of the Register Organizers in each of the Districts. Drs William Kearns, Angela Jones and Carol Martin were active participants and strong supporters of the scheme and without them many of the early difficulties would not have been overcome. More recently Mr David Pashley of the Regional Health Authority provided the inspiration, and the initial funding, to undertake the present exercise.

We thank Dr David Preston for his considerable assistance in managing the data files produced by each of the districts.

The initial software for the Register was written by Mr Ray Darker to whom we are grateful.

Acknowledgements

It is ironic that at this stage in the development of services for the care of people with mental handicaps, many of the Registers within the Region are being abandoned or revised to the point that an exercise such as this will be difficult to repeat. We earnestly hope that the management decisions to save money by disturbing an established and proven method of collecting data about this group of people will not ultimately result in a deterioration of services and increasing burdens on their families.

Preface

Until very recently, people with learning disabilities were referred to as people with mental handicaps. The change in terminology arose from a feeling that 'mental handicap' was prejudicial. It had tended to become a term of abuse, it was disliked by some of the people affected and was confused with mental illness. A change in terminology was also reflective of a general change in attitude towards those affected, specifically an appreciation that their quality of life might be improved by accommodating them within the community rather than isolating them in large specialist institutions. Interestingly, in the latest version of the International Classification of Disease (ICD 10) the definition of the term 'learning disabilities' specifically excludes intellectual deficit. Throughout this book the term 'mental handicap' is used because all the data were collected using that term.

The unifying characteristic of people with learning disabilities (mental handicap) is an intellectual deficit. In addition to their primary intellectual deficit most of those affected have either significant physical disabilities or behavioural problems, or both. A high proportion also have some form of sensory deficit. The incidence of concurrent chronic illness that requires regular medical supervision is high. Neither 'mental handicap' nor 'learning disabilities' give a clear indication of the complexities of their problems or their need for life long care.

The national policy in the United Kingdom to provide care within the 'community' and for a phased closure of the large mental handicap hospitals was developed during the 1960s and 1970s. At that time little population data was available to assess the real size of the problem, the needs of affected individuals or give a clear idea of their potential. About twelve years ago, the Health Authority serving most of the centre of London (Kensington and Chelsea and Westminster) realized that they had very little data on which to plan future services. It was decided to create and maintain a Register of all the people with mental handicaps to whom they had a responsibility. The Register was designed to assist in the planning of services for individual people, help in the evaluation of services and as a resource for research. It was apparent that these functions could not be met with a simple list of names, addresses and ages, thus from the outset data on the abilities and disabilities of individuals, and their living skills were included in the Register data set. Over the years other Registers have been developed and maintained throughout the North West Thames Region. In 1989 it was decided to aggregate the data from these Registers in order to gain an overview of the situation in a large population (about 8% of the population of England and Wales). This book is based on analyses of the collated data.

The work on the Registers was carried out with the conviction that people with mental handicaps and their families are a group for whom long-term planning is appropriate, necessary and, with information, relatively simple. Affected individuals and their families need an adequate volume, variety and quality of provision if they are not to suffer. To many people involved in day-to-day care, the contents of this book may appear to be detached, to others many of the findings may be obvious. We make no apology for finding and stating the obvious. We have tried to emphasize the complexities of the issues and the problems encountered in caring for this group in different situations, in the belief that a clear understanding is essential to promote the development of the correct quantity and quality of services. Sadly, even detailed information cannot guarantee that there will not be a decline in services in the new competitive environment of health and social care provision. The development and maintenance of a high standard of care requires a long-term commitment of resources and a continuing sensitivity to the needs of all those concerned. The fact that many of the Registers that provided data for this investigation are no longer being maintained bodes ill for the future.

During the period of operation of the Register there have been many administrative changes – the managerial structure of the National Health Service has changed twice, there have been boundary changes and the responsibility for the care of people with mental handicaps has been transferred from the NHS to the Social Service departments of the Local Government Authorities. Today there is great anxiety about the future of services for people with learning disabilities. The optimism of the early 1980s has disappeared within a maze of managerial hierarchies, ill-defined responsibilities, confused financial arrangements and a reduction in the real amount of money available to provide services. The needs of many, particularly those with multiple handicaps, are being neglected. Neither people with learning disabilities nor their families carry much political influence but this should not mean that they lose out in the modern welfare state. We hope that the contents of this book will promote understanding, initiate informed debate and ultimately play some part in achieving a better quality of life for people with learning disabilities.

Richard Farmer
Jenifer Rohde
Ben Sacks

1

Introduction

The terminology used to describe peple with primary mental handicaps has been subject to controversy and change since the nineteenth century. Although the current terminology in the UK is 'people with learning disabilities', the older term is used here. 'Mental handicap' remains the term favoured by the majority of parents of children with mental handicaps, and by the majority of the doctors directly involved in their care (Nursey et al., 1990).

In all societies, some people are mentally handicapped; because of their intellectual limitations they find it difficult to compete on equal terms with others in their communities. This has always been the situation. There are now a number of strategies for reducing the incidence of mental handicaps through immunization of women of childbearing age against diseases likely to cause congenital abnormalities (e.g., rubella); genetic counselling (e.g. fragile X syndrome); antenatal screening and selective abortion (e.g., chromosomal abnormalities); improved antenatal, intranatal, postnatal and infant care (Pueschel and Mulick 1990).

Despite these efforts, it is inevitable that some individuals continue to be affected. In recent years the prevalence of mental handicap has changed little; although many of the problems that caused mental handicap in the past have been eliminated or controlled, new problems have arisen. Characteristically, people with mental handicaps have difficulty surviving on their own. There is no indication that the problems faced by such people will be any less in time to come. Indeed, their problems may become more difficult to manage because of the increasing complexity and competitive nature of society, and the fact that intellectual achievement is now highly valued in all societies. The challenge is to create an environment in which people with mental handicaps can attain their maximum potential, and where they and their families have the best quality of life.

The performance of people with mental handicaps is affected by many factors other than their intellectual deficit. For example, their mobility, continence, sensory functioning, and ability to communicate all influence behaviour and social functioning.

The broad group of people recognized as having mental handicaps range from those who are physically normal with a mild intellectual deficit and few or no behavioural problems, to those who are multiply handicapped and whose existence depends upon the availability of expert and intensive care. The heterogeneous nature of people described as mentally handicapped calls for a diversity of care provisions sensitive to their own individual needs and to those of their families.

Before the twentieth century

It is not easy to say how people with mental handicaps were cared for in the eighteenth and early nineteenth centuries. Tracing the development of formal-care systems is relatively easy, but does not tell the whole story. We can only guess at the number who lived at home with their relatives.

Scientific concern with 'idiots' grew in Europe and the US at the end of the eighteenth century as an offshoot of the growth of 'psychological medicine', and interest in the care of those with sensory impairments. The treatment of the 'Wild Boy of Aveyron' was a notable milestone (Adams, 1971).

Advances in psychological medicine in the nineteenth century enabled people with mental handicaps to be distinguished from those who were blind, deaf, mentally ill, or who were senile. By the turn of the century, several developments had combined to identify people with low levels of intellect as a 'problem group' who should be provided for appropriately. These developments included the increasing concern with eugenics – the fear that selective breeding would increase the numbers of 'inferior' members of society; and the development of universal, compulsory elementary education.

The eugenic fear arose from a concern that class conflict would spill over into violence and civil war, and became a constant preoccupation among European ruling groups. This fear received a further impetus as nations drawn into conflict (e.g. Britain at the time of the Boer War) found that many of their young men were deemed unfit for military service. 'Mental defectives' were perceived as extremely fertile, and a threat to racial quality.

Universal education brought with it the necessity to examine the physical and mental abilities of all children. The solution to 'feeble-minded' children was seen as segregation and education in special classes (Alaszewski, 1988).

The era of institutions

Following the 1908 Royal Commission and the 1913 Mental Deficiency Act, mentally defective and mentally ill people were segregated as a solution to their perceived threat to established society. The main alternative to that policy, sterilization, raised ethical and practical problems. Implementation of segregation, delayed by the First World War, went ahead in the 1920s. In 1929, the Wood Committee considered that about one-third of the 300 000 mental defectives in England and Wales would require segregation (Alaszewski, 1988). Adams (1971) charts a similar process in the US with the growth of segregated institutions for both children and adults, but an estimate in 1915 suggested that only 10% of the 'feeble-minded' were in institutions.

Many of the British institutions had extensive grounds, and were supported by their own farms and market gardens, on which the able residents worked. They were sited in the country away from the main centres of population, often at great distances from the communities from which the residents originated. Many of them are still in use today, some with only minimal modernization. Legislation required that residents had to be certified and, once admitted, many remained for life.

Into the community

Formal schemes of 'community care' have been in existence for almost as long as the large mental handicap institutions. In the last years of the nineteenth century, a system of 'scattered homes' was created in Sheffield and in parts of London where, as Ayers (1971) describes:

> A few ordinary dwelling houses were ... acquired in Pentonville, Fulham, Wandsworth and Peckham. In each of these, 12 to 20 children were grouped according to age and sex. They resided in the homes in the care of foster parents and were encouraged to lead as normal a life as possible.

The children attended the local special schools for the handicapped.

It is over the past two decades, however, that attitudes towards people with mental handicaps have changed most rapidly in Western countries.

In the UK in 1957, a Royal Commission on the law relating to mental illness and mental handicap recommended that the existing formal legal framework should be abandoned in favour of more flexible provision. It proposed that the universal practice of certification with subsequent formal review should be abandoned. Where possible, admission was to be informal, and when formal certification was necessary, regular review was to be mandatory. It was also proposed that facilities for care in the community should be encouraged and publicly funded in order to reduce the dependency on large, antiquated hospitals, and to offer a better quality of life. Many of the recommendations of the Royal Commission were reflected in the Mental Health Act (1959).

The changes achieved by the late 1960s fell short of early expectations. In 1969 the secretary of state for social services commissioned a study of the services for and the needs of the mentally handicapped. The report of the study was published in 1971 by the Department of Health and Social Security and the Welsh Office as 'Better Services for the Mentally Handicapped'. It recommended a number of changes, including:

- Services should be developed to facilitate early diagnosis, to enable comprehensive assessments of the future needs of the handicapped person and his or her family (Para. 131).
- Research should be promoted into the causes of mental handicap and its prevention, with a view to expanding counselling services to at-risk parents (Para. 126).
- Active education and training programmes should be developed for the mentally handicapped (Para. 154).
- The promotion of a framework to support the families, to include counselling and the encouragement of local parent-support groups (Para. 139).
- The introduction of a wide range of types of residential and other services in every area, to give scope for the particular needs of individuals to be met (Para. 158).
- A change in the philosophy and environment of institutions to bring about a 'home-like' atmosphere (Para. 184).
- Greater co-ordination of services (including voluntary services) with the objective of building a sense of partnership among the care providers (Para. 264).
- The avoidance of unnecessary segregation of the mentally handicapped with the objective of their achieving a more integrated way of life (Para. 39).
- The continued use of improved hospital services by those for whom it is needed (Para. 238).
- Greater emphasis on staff training and retraining in order that the personnel would be equipped to provide the recommended new style of care. (Para. 231).

The report set targets for the provision of services, which were to be based on 'norms' for particular population sizes. These norms were estimated from data obtained from three surveys in Wessex, Newcastle, and Camberwell (Kushlick *et al.*, 1973; Neligan *et al.*, 1974; Wing, 1972). The authors of 'Better Services for the Mentally Handicapped' acknowledged the limitations of their 'tentative and provisional' figures and stated that 'Any estimates made now as a basis for planning services will need to be adjusted in the light of experience and further research'.

It was proposed that the numbers of people in mental handicap hospitals should be reduced by transferring the more able into 'community' settings, and by preventing inappropriate admissions. It was also thought to be essential to refurbish and upgrade the hospitals. The reduced number of places in hospital was to be balanced by an increase in the number of places in day and residential care in the 'community', and by building new, small, hospital units.

In response to the White Paper, the government appointed a Committee for Enquiry into Mental Handicap Nursing and Care (*The Jay Report*, 1979). It identified three broad sets of principles, which in combination underpinned their thinking:

a) Mentally handicapped people have a right to enjoy normal patterns of life within the community.

b) Mentally handicapped people have a right to be treated as individuals.

c) Mentally handicapped people will require additional help from the communities in which they live and from professional services if they are to develop their maximum potential as individuals.

The Committee expanded on the implications of their philosophy by suggesting where people with mental handicaps should live, in what type of environment, and how services should be organized. Their message was:

... that individuals with mental handicaps should have as much autonomy and control over their lives as was consistent with their ability, that they should live within their own 'communities' rather than being geographically and socially separated, and that as far as possible the provision of medical and social care should be through the generic services.

An important criticism of the Report is that it tended to regard persons with mental handicaps as a group whose needs could be met within a single model of care, and whose rights could be universally defined.

The reality is that people with mental handicaps comprise a diverse group with a vast range of physical, sensory, behavioural, intellectual, and other problems. In particular, the needs of those with multiple handicaps, and their families, and the needs of those with severe behavioural disorders were not fully considered in the Report. The notion that the psychiatric, neurological, and medical needs of this group of people could be managed within the generic medical services was assumed rather than demonstrated. The logistical problems for someone caring for a multiply handicapped person, who would have to escort him or her to many clinics within the standard health care model, was not addressed. Furthermore, the clinical implications of attending many specialists was not considered.

In 1975 the secretary of state for health and social services set up the National Development Group, which was essentially a policy group to advise on the implementation of better services for the mentally handicapped. For a short time it coexisted with another organization called the National Development Team for Mentally Handicapped People (NDT). The function of this group was to visit hospitals and advise authorities on practice. Even though the NDT had few statutory powers, it influenced the nature and pace of changes in this field.

The last decade has seen an increasing emphasis on locally-based support, management, and care. Many hospital beds and a few complete hospitals have been closed (Wing, 1989). Admission and readmission rates have fallen in many parts of the country; however, in some areas, following an initial fall, admissions have risen, as has the number of occupied beds. There have been some developments in the provision of residential and day-care facilities both by the statutory authorities and voluntary organizations.

The numbers of inpatients in designated mental handicap hospitals in successive years are shown in Table 1.1. The fall in numbers began in the early 1970s. By 1989 (the last national figures available) inpatients had fallen to about 50% of the 1964 numbers (Figure 1.1). The indications are that the numbers of hospital inpatients have continued to fall since 1989.

First-ever admissions to mental handicap hospitals in England started falling from the late 1960s (Figure 1.2). The reduction in the numbers of children and young people admitted was the most dramatic, from about 3500 to about

Table 1.1 Total numbers of inpatients in mental handicap hospitals in England (1000s)

1964	56.1
1969	56.2
1974	48.2
1979	45.4
1984	38.4
1986	34.2
1989	27.7
1990	24.9 (provisional)

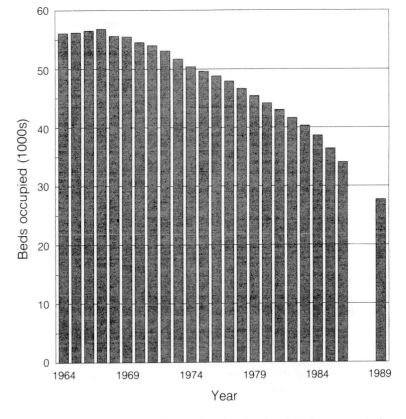

Figure 1.1 Mental handicap hospitals in England and Wales – occupied beds by year.

8

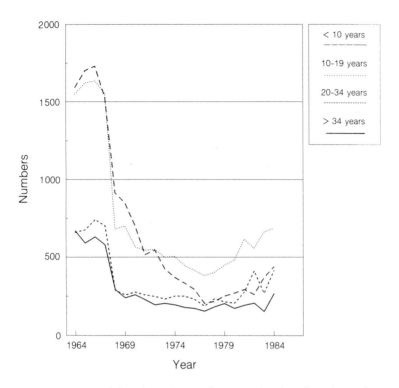

Figure 1.2 Mental handicap hospitals in England and Wales – first admissions by age group and year.

1000 per year. In the 1980s there was a modest rise in first admissions in all age groups. Since the early 1970s, the number of readmissions has risen (Figure 1.3). Readmissions now account for about 95% of all admissions to hospitals for people with mental handicaps.

This change in patterns of admission reflects a change in policy from regarding admission as a permanent solution, to one where the hospitals are expected to provide short-term care and only admit to long-term care the relatively few people who cannot be placed elsewhere. These observations indicate that the general threshold of admission has been raised. The declared objective of caring for the new generation

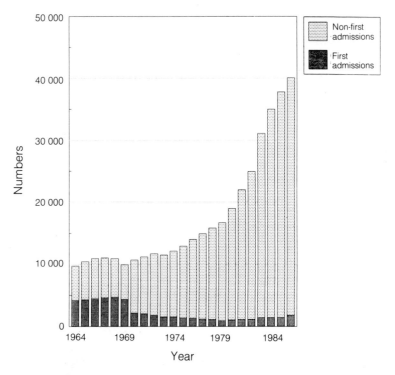

Figure 1.3 Mental handicap hospitals in England and Wales– admissions by year.

of people with mental handicaps out of hospital has been partially achieved – fewer people are now managed in hospital.

The above observations are confirmed by the trends in discharges according to length of stay (Figure 1.4). There has been little change in the number of discharges of people whose stay had been over three months. There is a massive increase in the numbers discharged within three months of admission. In short, part of the change has been to replace a 'closed door' with a 'revolving door'. This may be a beneficial change, but it appears to fall far short of the aims of the Committees that reported in the late 1960s and early 1970s.

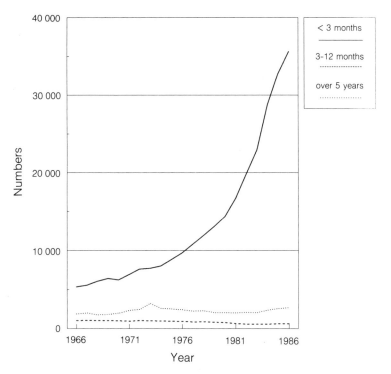

Figure 1.4 Mental handicap hospitals in England and Wales – discharges and deaths by duration of stay.

The current situation

The recent changes and developments, although generally beneficial, have produced a new set of problems:

The policy of hospital bed closures and avoidance of admission has resulted in a new cohort of young adults living at home, who in previous generations would have been admitted to hospital. There is a limit to the time that an individual family, however well supported, will be able to provide care. There is a clear need for a range of residential options.

The development of non-hospital day facilities (social education centres, day centres, etc.) has failed to keep pace with the increase in the numbers and change in the range in

11

ability of people with mental handicaps living in the community. In particular, the social education centres and day centres are sometimes reluctant to accept people who have combinations of physical, psychiatric, and behavioural problems.

As the more able have been discharged, the residual hospital population consists of an ageing and more dependent group requiring more intensive care and supervision (Farmer *et al.*, 1990).

A fragmented approach to community care, largely involving unskilled personnel drawn from a wide range of employing authorities, might result in a deterioration in the quality of care.

The financial implications of past changes and future plans have not yet been fully assessed. Money is made available to community services, through the 'dowry' system, whereby local authorities or health authorities who accept the residents of long-stay hospitals for resettlement in their community become entitled to a significant proportion of the notional capital and revenue that would have been spent had that person remained in hospital. However, there may be insufficient funds for those who, in earlier days, would have been admitted to long-term care. There is a lack of appreciation of the scale of finance that is required for 'community' care, especially for the multiply handicapped, and the need for day services is often forgotten. The situation is further complicated by the balance of financial responsibility between the health service and the social services being ill-defined.

Counting the numbers

It is only recently that attempts have been made to count the numbers of people with mental handicaps. Even current estimates may still be subject to a degree of error; however, the creation of comprehensive registers (Fryers, 1984; Cubbon and Malin, 1985) has added greatly to the precision with which estimates can be made, and has helped to rationalize the planning of services. The registers of the NW Thames regional health authorities (RHA) (Figure 1.5) provide a unique opportunity for the appraisal of recent changes. Detailed analysis of these data can be used to develop an understanding of the current situation and may suggest strategies for the future.

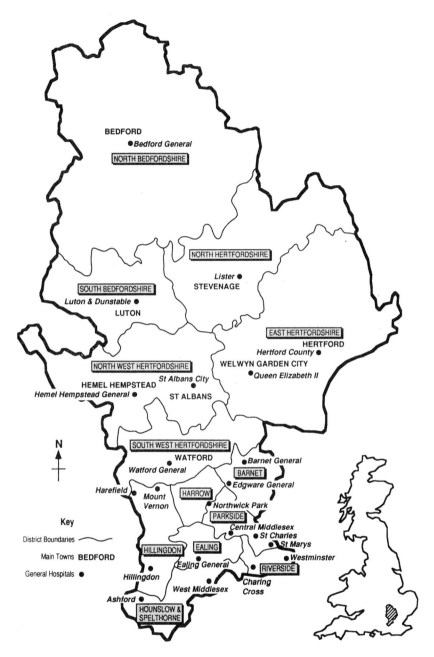

Figure 1.5 NW Thames RHA.

13

2

The register system

In the past, the absence of reliable data on the incidence and prevalence of people with mental handicaps has limited the precision with which services could be planned and evaluated. The effect is that much planning has been based on crude population 'norms' for service provision. Planning on this basis takes little or no account of the social and demographic differences between populations, and the variations in the facilities required by individuals within the broad category known as 'mental handicap'. The lack of systematic population-based data has also restricted the type of research that could be undertaken to establish the causes of handicap, factors that affect its severity in individuals, and the rational development of preventive programmes.

There have been several attempts in the past to maintain large population-based information systems on people with mental handicaps – Sheffield (Martindale, 1976); Salford (Fryers, 1984); and Camberwell (Wing, 1972). The pioneering work of Kushlick *et al.* (1973) provided an invaluable framework within which to collect data, and to make broad individual assessments in this field.

During the review of the National Development Team's report on its progress in the late 1970s, the Kensington and Chelsea and Westminster Area Health Authority (KCWAHA) realized it did not know how many mentally handicapped people was its responsibility; nor were the severities of handicap, the level of concurrent disabilities, or places of residence known. In effect, the only basis for planning was national 'norms'. This was thought to be an unsatisfactory situation.

Although the first response was to conduct a prevalence survey, that idea was abandoned in favour of developing and maintaining a register of all the people who were either mentally handicapped, or who were using or might use services for the mentally handicapped to whom the Authority had a responsibility.

On the whole, people with mental handicaps are identifiable at a young age and remain handicapped throughout their lives; therefore, a well-maintained, comprehensive database should make it possible to plan for specific individuals and groups.

The methodology of the original register was developed in the Academic Department of Community Medicine of Westminster Medical School (Farmer and Rohde, 1983), which became fully operational in 1982. A register for the population that had previously been covered by KCWAHA has been maintained by the Department ever since.

The registration and assessment of all the individuals with mental handicaps was usually made by the person mainly responsible for the care of the individual, irrespective of their professional background; in some cases this was a parent. In cases where the principal carer was unable or unwilling to make the assessment, the person next most closely involved was approached. The type of data that are collected, and regularly updated, on all the identified individuals with mental handicaps falls into the following five groups:

1. Personal identification and characteristics (name, date of birth, sex, marital condition, address, next-of-kin, and so on).
2. Residential placement and daytime occupation.
3. Nature and cause of the primary handicap (causal diagnosis, complicating illnesses and disabilities, IQ).
4. Physical abilities and disabilities (mobility, continence, sensory function, communication, and so on).
5. Behavioural problems (attention-seeking, self-injury, and so on).

(The full data set is shown in Appendix A.)

The register system

In the mid-1980s, the NW Thames RHA sponsored similar register systems throughout the region. It financed the installation and maintenance of the systems, and subsidized staff in each of the districts. It was believed that the maintenance of a common system throughout the region would encourage good planning at district level, and would provide a framework to assess progress. Because all districts were using a common format, the region would be able to collate the data to provide a region-wide view of people with mental handicaps.

The Registers of People with Mental Handicaps have now been maintained in the districts for at least five years. During that time it has been the policy of the local health and social services authorities to discharge as many people as possible from hospitals to places in the community; to encourage care in the community; and to enable the closure of the old mental handicap hospitals.

In spring 1989 data from the following registers were merged to form a regional database:

- South Bedfordshire (S. Beds)
- Hillingdon (Hill'don)
- Brent
- Hounslow and Spelthorne (H. and S.)
- East Hertfordshire (E. Herts)
- North Hertfordshire (N. Herts)
- Hammersmith and Fulham (H'smith)
- South West Hertfordshire (S.W. Herts)
- Kensington and Chelsea and Westminster (KCW)
- Harrow.

3

Prevalence

Introduction

The mental handicap registers which formed the basis of this investigation were established for service-planning purposes. People eligible for registration were defined as those who used one or more of the specialist services for the mentally handicapped, or who were thought likely to require such services in the future, and who were the responsibility of one of the participating health districts. The merged registers of the NW Thames RHA, which includes 13 districts, provided information on 6625 individuals meeting the above inclusion criteria. Table 3.1 lists the participating health districts; the name of the register covering each district; the numbers of cases on each register; the population served; and the crude prevalence rate of people with mental handicaps.

The KCW register had the highest crude registration rate – the number of registrations divided by the total estimated population. The NW Hertfordshire register, serving the NW Hertfordshire and North Hertfordshire districts, had the lowest rate.

The crude registration rates distort the real prevalence of people with mental handicaps for several reasons:

In some districts there was an under-identification of people with mental handicaps; moreover, the degree of under-identification tended to vary across age groups. In some cases the authorities were unaware of the existence of some of the

Table 3.1 Cases on registers and populations served

Register authority	District Health Authority	Cases on register	Pop. (1000s)	Crude rate per 1000
Brent	Parkside (N.)	524	254.9	2.06
E. Herts	E. Herts	852	292.7	2.91
H'smith	Riverside (W.)	431	150.9	2.86
Harrow	Harrow	335	201.7	1.66
Hill'don	Hillingdon	667	232.1	2.87
H. and S.	H'slow and S.	622	285.8	2.18
KCW	Riverside (E.)	924	137.5	
	and Parkside (S.)		122.6	3.55
N. Herts	N.W. Herts	393	261.7	
	and N. Herts		186.6	0.88
S.W. Herts	S.W. Herts	593	245.1	2.42
S. Beds	N. Beds and	1284	242.0	
	S. Beds		274.7	2.49
All		6625	2888.3	2.29

affected individuals. Some of the careworkers felt that formal registration might prejudice people's future development. A few parents were unwilling to accept their child's handicap, and explicitly refused consent for registration.

In some districts the people responsible for registration failed to update their records with sufficient regularity to be certain that all people who were eligible had been included.

It was the policy of some authorities not to register any children before a particular age – in some cases this was five years, and in others it was thirteen years. The rationale for excluding children varied. Sometimes it was felt that formal registration – labelling – would prejudice the social development and integration of the child, whatever his or her level of disability. Some groups held the view that mental handicap could not be diagnosed with precision until a child reached a certain age – somewhat surprisingly, some paediatricians held this opinion, even in cases of Down's syndrome and other chromosomal abnormalities that are closely associated with an intellectual deficit. From the age breakdown of those registered

Table 3.2 Ages of persons registered on each Register

Register authority	Nk	0–4	5–14	15–29	30–44	45–64	>65	All
Brent	1	0	24	219	161	86	33	524
E. Herts	22	3	115	337	198	130	47	852
H'smith	4	0	0	152	126	104	43	431
Harrow	1	0	11	96	109	98	19	335
Hill'don	0	0	62	237	218	123	27	667
H. and S.	12	1	71	231	160	114	33	622
KCW	4	1	73	293	238	194	121	924
N. Herts	0	0	75	169	113	32	4	393
S.W. Herts	1	3	50	168	214	123	33	593
S. Beds	1	14	185	493	334	185	72	1284
All	46	22	666	2395	1871	1189	434	6625

Table 3.3 Age-specific case registration rates (1000s)

Register authority	5–14	15–29	30–44	45–64	>65
Brent	0.81	3.29	3.04	1.60	0.97
E. Herts	3.03	4.88	3.17	1.91	1.25
H'smith	0.00	3.81	3.68	3.57	1.75
Harrow	0.45	2.10	2.55	2.24	0.59
Hill'don	2.23	4.22	4.66	2.36	0.79
H. and S.	2.06	3.45	2.65	1.75	0.81
KCW	3.33	3.07	3.40	2.97	2.51
N. Herts	1.26	1.63	1.19	0.31	0.07
S.W. Herts	1.62	3.04	4.23	2.17	0.90
S. Beds	2.58	3.86	3.02	1.70	1.18

(Table 3.2) it is clear that the registration of children is at best sporadic.

The denominator population used in the calculation of the crude prevalence rate was distorted by the way in which individuals were assigned as the responsibility of a particular authority. People living in their family homes were deemed to be the responsibility of the authority covering that geographical area. Those in residential care were the responsibility of the authority covering the area in which they or their

19

next-of-kin were living at the time of admission to residential care. Many of the people in hospital had been resident for many years, some for over 50 years. At the time of admission, the size of the local population from which they were drawn was significantly different from its current level. This is most pronounced in Central London, where the population halved between 1940 and 1990. Thus, the apparent prevalence of elderly people with mental handicaps in, for example, KCW or in Hammersmith and Fulham is remarkably high (Table 3.3).

Estimation of true prevalence

As registration was known to be incomplete, the real prevalence of people with mental handicaps within the populations served by the registers could not be calculated directly. Among the adults, some adjustment had to be made for incomplete registration; children presented a particular problem since so little information was available. Therefore, it was necessary to use the recorded numbers within a model to estimate the true age-specific prevalence.

The exact age of 6579 (99.3%) individuals on the registers was known. Among them there were only 22 children under the age of five years, the majority of whom were on the Bedfordshire register. Most registers had remarkably few children aged 5–14 years. Additionally, the crude registration rate in North Hertfordshire was atypically low, and was thought to have been the result of gross under-registration. In view of these observations, it was decided to omit North Hertfordshire and children under the age of 15 years from the data set used to model the population prevalence.

Modelling methods

Assuming no net migration in the population, the number of mentally handicapped people alive at a given age is determined by the number of births in a particular year and their cumulative mortality – how many have died up to the year of observation. For example, if there were 100 births of affected babies in 1981, the number of affected individuals age 10 years in 1991 would be 100 less the number who had died between birth and 1991. It follows that the proportion of the population of a given age who are mentally handicapped is determined by the proportion of the population born with mental handicaps in a particular year and their differential mortality – the difference between the death rate among people with mental handicaps and the rest of the population – up to the year of observation, again assuming no net migration of either population.

Live births of children with mental handicaps are not recorded separately from all births. Separate national death rates for people with mental handicaps are not available; it is therefore impossible to estimate the size of the mentally handicapped population using a straightforward survival model.

Mortality among people with mental handicaps is higher than that of the general population (Eyman, 1990; O'Brien *et al.*, 1991; Richards and Siddiqui, 1980).

In order to establish the proportion of the population who have a mental handicap at each year of age, it is essential to know both the number of handicapped individuals and the size of the population from which they were drawn. The total resident population of the districts involved in the investigation

Table 3.4 Population of NW Thames RHA compared with England and Wales (1988)

	England and Wales		NW Thames RHA*	
Age	Numbers (millions)	%	Numbers (millions)	%
<1	0.686	1.36	0.039	1.44
1–4	2.602	5.16	0.141	5.23
5–14	6.121	12.15	0.317	11.79
15–29	11.837	23.49	0.654	24.35
30–44	10.418	20.67	0.580	21.59
45–59	8.187	16.25	0.442	16.45
60–64	2.607	5.17	0.130	4.84
65–74	4.484	8.90	0.216	8.04
>74	3.452	6.85	0.168	6.26
Total	50.393	100.00	2.686	100.00

*Participating districts

21

was 2.69 million – about 5.3% of the population of England and Wales (Table 3.4). The distribution of the population of the participating districts according to broad age groups did not differ significantly from that of England and Wales (Chi^2 = 0.0024; df = 8; NS). Unfortunately the distribution of the district populations according to exact year of age was not available. In view of the close agreement between the age-group distribution of the national population and that of the parent population, the exact age distribution of the national population was used in the calculations that follow.

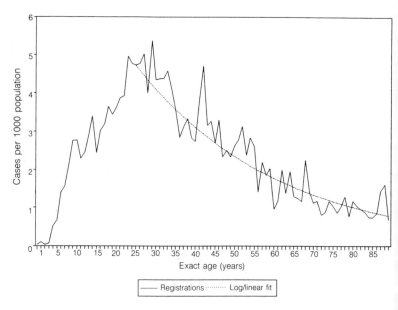

Figure 3.1 Proportion of the population registered as having mental handicaps.

Figure 3.1 shows the proportion of the estimated total population who have a mental handicap and are covered by the registers. Because of under-registration among children and young people, the proportions up to the age of 20 are meaningless. The proportions relating to people over the age of 24 fit a log-linear curve (r^2 = 0.85). The proportion affected appears to decline from five to one per 100 between 20–75 years. If it is assumed that the birth incidence of mental handicap has remained more or less constant during this century – there are no data with which to explore the validity of this assumption – then the changes in the proportion of the population who are mentally handicapped across age groups is explained by their differential mortality.

The hypothesis that the ratio of the age-specific death rates among people with mental handicaps to those of the general population follow an exponential decay curve can be tested in two ways.

First, the KCW register has accumulated data over a 12-year period, and it was therefore possible to calculate the death rates among those registered over the period 1985–90. These rates, together with the national death rates for the same period, are shown in Table 3.5. There is a negative exponential relationship between the two.

Second, Eyman (1990) studied the life expectancy of 99 543 people with 'developmental disabilities' in order to establish the life expectancy of people with profound handicaps. They presented detailed data on three groups of people, all with profound, severe, or suspected mental retardation. Individuals in group one were immobile, not toilet-trained and required tube feeding; those in group two were immobile, were not toilet-trained and were able to be fed by others; group three individuals were ambulatory, not toilet-trained and were able to be fed

Table 3.5 Average annual death rates (1985–90) of people with mental handicaps resident in KCW compared with all residents of England and Wales

| Age group | Deaths (1000s) | | Ratio MH national rates |
	Mental handicap	Total pop.	
15–24	4.98	0.56	8.89
25–34	5.12	0.67	7.67
35–44	5.83	1.41	4.13
45–54	12.61	3.86	3.27
55–64	45.45	11.47	3.87
65–74	39.26	30.16	1.30
75–84	81.83	73.27	1.11
85–94	283.02	153.83	1.85

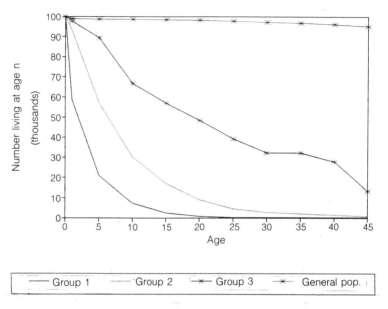

Figure 3.2 People with 'mental retardation' life table data.

by others. The data from Eyman's life tables together with life table data for the general population are shown in Figure 3.2.

The pattern of decline in the proportion of the population who are handicapped within the region is consistent with both of the above findings. Thus, it is not unreasonable to extrapolate the exponential distribution of the ratio of people with mental handicaps to the estimated total population by exact year of age (calculated from persons age 24–99 years) back to age 0 years. This yields an expected ratio across all ages.

The estimated numbers of people with handicaps is the product of the 'fitted' ratio and the estimated total population. Figure 3.3 shows the estimated numbers of people with mental handicaps within the populations covered by the registers, with the exception of NW Hertfordshire. The observed and estimated prevalence rates for people with mental handicaps, as defined by the criteria used in this investigation, are shown in Table 3.6. There is reasonably good agreement between the calculated and observed numbers of people over the age of 45 years. The agreement is satisfactory between the ages of 20–45 years. Among the younger people, the difference between the observed and expected numbers reflects under-registration. The overall calculated incidence of people with mental handicaps is 4.04 per 1000 living.

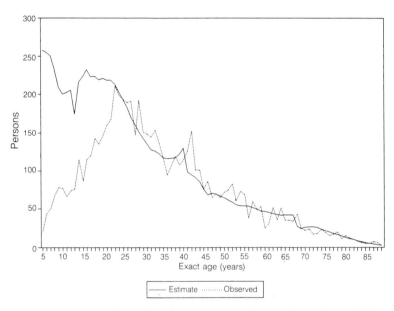

Figure 3.3 Estimated population of people with mental handicaps (NW Thames).

Table 3.6 Observed and estimated prevalence rates of people with mental handicaps

Age	Prevalence (1000s)	
	Observed	Estimated
5–14 years	2.22	7.34
15–29	4.07	5.18
30–44	3.65	3.40
45–64	2.22	2.09
>64	1.14	1.25
All >5	2.67	4.04

The degree of intellectual impairment (degree of mental handicap) was specified for 3804 individuals on the registers over the age of 15 years (that is 64.6% of all registered over the age of 15 years). The numbers in each group and percentages by age are shown in Table 3.7. The proportion who are severely handicapped decreases with age. This is likely to be the result of differential survival according to the degree of handicap and is consistent with the findings from Eyman (1990). If those on the registers for whom the degree of handicap is known are representative of all people with mental handicap on the registers, then the estimated population prevalence of people with an IQ of less than 50 (the usual designation for surveys of mental handicap) can be derived by deducting the proportion with 'Mild Mental Handicap' from the estimated prevalence rate of those requiring services for people with mental handicap. The derived estimates of the incidence of people with an IQ of less than 50 are shown in Table 3.8.

Table 3.7 Degree of intellectual impairment (handicap) of people registered over age 15 years ( ) = column %

	Age group				
Handicap	*15–29*	*30–44*	*45–64*	*>64*	*Total*
Mild	299	338	281	125	1043
(IQ 50–70)	(21.1)	(27.5)	(34.3)	(36.7)	(27.4)
Moderate	361	340	241	107	1049
(IQ 35–49)	(25.6)	(27.6)	(29.4)	(31.4)	(27.6)
Severe	618	473	256	103	1450
(IQ 20–34)	(43.8)	(38.4)	(31.2)	(30.2)	(38.1)
Profound	134	80	42	6	262
(IQ < 20)	(9.5)	(6.5)	(5.1)	(1.8)	(6.9)
All known	1412	1231	820	341	3804

Table 3.8 Estimates of population prevalence of IQs < 50

Age group	*Gross prevalence*	*IQ < 50*
15–29	5.18	4.08
30–44	3.40	2.63
45–64	2.09	1.37
65–74	1.25	0.79
All > 15	4.04	2.93

Table 3.9 Estimates of the incidence and prevalence of mental handicap in different populations (1000s)

Country	Group	Cases/1000
Northern Ireland (Mallon *et al.*, 1991)	Age 20–29: IQ < 50 Eastern and Northern HB Southern and Western HB	4.07–4.82 5.17–6.37
Northern Ireland (Elwood and Darragh 1981)	IQ < 50 1950–69 birth cohort	3.67
Italy (Bologna) (Benassi *et al.*, 1990)	IQ < 50: Age 6–14 Males Females All	4.2 2.5 3.4
Hungary (Czeizel *et al.*, 1990)	IQ < 50 School age	3.0
Denmark (Andersen *et al.*, 1990)	Birth cohort at age 4 'Mental Retardation'	2.9
Sweden (Gothenburg) (Hagberg *et al.*, 1987)	IQ < 50: Age 8–12 IQ < 50: Age 14–18	3.0 3.3
Sweden (Hagberg *et al.*, 1983)	IQ < 50 School age	3.0
Sweden (Gostason, 1985)	IQ < 50 All males IQ < 50 All females	4.0 3.7
Spain (Jaen) (Delgado, 1989)	IQ < 50	4.04
Spain (Galicia) (Diaz-Fernandez, 1988)	Total population IQ < 50	3.4
New Zealand (Joyce *et al.*, 1988)	IQ < 50 Age 10	4.35
Latvia (Vilnyus) (Puras, 1987)	Severe mental retardation Age 4–13	3.1
Canada (McQueen *et al.*, 1987)	Major mental retardation	3.65
Canada (Baird and Sadovnick, 1985)	All levels retardation Age 15–29	7.7
Northern Finland (Rantakallio and von Wendt, 1986)	IQ < 50 Age 14	7.4
British Columbia (Herbst and Baird, 1983)	Non-specific mental retardation: Age 15–29	4.4

The estimated prevalence of people with severe or profound mental handicap (IQ < 50) over the age of 15 in this population is 2.93 per 1000. Fryers (1984) estimated of incidence of severe and profound mental handicap (IQ < 50) in England and Wales as 5.4 per 1000 live births and a prevalence as 3–4 per 1000 total population, including children under the age of 15 years. Elliott *et al*. (1981) found a prevalence among children age 5–14 in Oxfordshire (England) of 3.9 per 1000. Similar prevalences have been reported from other countries (Tables 3.9).

Gostason (1985) estimated the age specific prevalence of mental handicap in a Swedish county. He used register data supplemented by some information collected during the course of a population survey. Prevalence fell with age both for severe (IQ < 50) and moderate mental handicap (IQ > 50 but < 70). His estimated rates of severe handicap are a little higher than those in the present study (Table 3.10).

Table 3.10 Prevalence of mental handicap in a Swedish county (Gostason, 1985)

	Mental handicap		
Age	*Severe*	*Moderate*	*All*
20–29	6.4	5.3	11.6
30–39	3.7	5.0	8.7
40–49	3.3	4.6	7.9
50–59	2.2	5.2	7.4

Limitations of the estimate

The above estimates assume that the proportion of babies born between 1969–89 who were affected with mental handicaps was similar to those of earlier birth cohorts and that patterns of mortality have not changed. Both of these assumptions may be challenged – for example, it is possible that the introduction of systematic prenatal screening and elective abortion may have reduced the incidence of some congenital abnormalities associated with mental handicap. On the other hand, improvements in neonatal care would have increased the survival rate of some other groups and an increase in maternal age would have tended to increase incidence.

Developments in medical care available in the post-neonatal period would be expected to decrease mortality (Baird and Sadovnick, 1985; Simila *et al.*, 1986). The result of these changes could well be that they had no net effect on the incidence of handicap – indeed changes in medical care (resulting in increased survival) has led to an increase in the prevalence of mental handicap (O'Brien *et al.*, 1991; McLoughlin, 1988; Wolf and Wright, 1987). Taking all factors into consideration, we believe that the estimated incidence rates can be used as reasonable guides to the numbers of people for whom facilities should be planned.

Broad estimates of the prevalence of severe mental handicap have limitations when used for planning services for affected individuals. The type of facilities required to care for individuals in this group is determined as much by their behaviour, physical disabilities, and social circumstances as it is by their intellectual deficit. Therefore, forecasting the type of facilities that should be provided presents a complex problem. In this monograph we show that people with mental handicaps form a diverse group. Apart from their underlying mental handicaps, a high proportion are affected with physical disabilities, concurrent physical and psychiatric illness, and many have severe behavioural problems.

No single model of care will suffice for this group of people. A wide range of facilities, both residential and otherwise, are now provided and will need to be provided in the future. If those on the registers are representative of all affected with mental handicaps, and if the next generation, those now aged 0–15 years, is similar to the present, then it can be confidently predicted that about one-quarter will be highly dependent – either because of their underlying mental handicap, or because of other handicaps and disabilities, or both.

In earlier generations these people would have been cared for in long-stay mental handicap hospitals. The community schemes that have been developed in the last two decades have proved successful for many people with mental handicaps (Locker *et al.*, 1984; Cattermole *et al*, 1988; Jahoda *et al*, 1990, Fleming and Stenfert Kroese, 1990). In recent years, for many people, the main responsibility has remained with their families in recent years. Even if it is agreed that the mainstay of care should be the biological family, there will be a proportion for whom this option does not exist. This may be due to death or infirmity of the natural parents, or their inability or unwillingness to provide care or other reasons. For those who remain with their families, support from the social, education, and health services will be required.

4

Places of residence

Until about 20 years ago, the majority of people with mental handicaps who did not live with their families were cared for in hospitals managed by the NHS authorities. Since the 1960s there has been a greater emphasis on caring for people outside hospital settings, and attempts have been made to avoid hospital admissions. Moreover, it has been the policy to discharge people from hospitals into alternative accommodation in the community. Most of the hospitals have reduced the number of available beds, and some have closed completely.

Within the registers, the place of residence is classified as follows.

Family home

This refers to the individual's family home, in which people with mental handicaps are looked after by their parents or siblings. People who are living independently, in their own homes, without the support of a non-handicapped relative are excluded from this category. Of the people on the registers, currently 2412 (41.6%) live in their family home.

Hospital

This refers exclusively to hospitals for the mentally handicapped are managed by the NHS. Their sizes vary from about 70 residents to over 1000. The costs are borne by the NHS budget. Of the people on the registers, 1494 (25.8%) currently live in hospital.

Local Authority (LA) homes or hostels

These are institutions owned by the local government authorities and managed through their social services departments. Usually these homes are designed to provide accommodation for 5–30 people. They are funded by the LA through local taxes (rates or community charge) supplemented by monies paid directly from the central government department of social security. Of the people on the registers, 627 (10.8%) currently live in LA accommodation.

Private and/or voluntary homes (P/V)

These are either owned by charities, for example, the Royal Society for Mentally Handicapped Children and Adults (MENCAP), religious orders and so on, or are privately owned and run for profit. They are not necessarily located within the same geographical area as that from which the residents are drawn, nor are they always close to the place of residence of relatives. They vary a great deal in the range of facilities and standards of care, some offering a complete and almost self-sufficient community, others simply providing sheltered accommodation and food. The individual residents are paid for in part by the LAs from which the person was admitted, and in part from central funds through the social security system. Of the people on the registers, 608 (10.5%) currently live in P/V accommodation.

Foster homes

These are used for some people with mental handicaps, mostly children and young adults. Families are paid to accept the handicapped person into their own homes and provide complete care for them. The costs are met from central and local government funds. Of the people on the registers, 61 (1.1%) are currently in foster homes.

Residential schools

There are two types of school. Some are owned by the local government authorities, and others by private or religious foundations. They are specialized boarding schools that provide education and residential facilities during term times, the pupils usually returning to their families during the vacations. Residential schools may not be an option for individuals who do not have alternative accommodation during vacations.

Residential schools normally provide for people up to the age of 19 years. Those with severe handicaps – either mental or physical, or both – tend to be excluded except by a few highly specialized establishments. Of the children on the registers, 85 (12.7%) attend residential schools. (The percentage of children on the registers who attend special residential schools must be viewed with caution since there is a substantial under-registration of children generally; it is more likely that a child who is attending one of these schools will be known to the register organizers, than a child who is not using any residential provision outside the family.)

Independents

Some 181 (3.1%) of people with mental handicaps live 'independently'. This way of living is currently being encouraged by the authorities. The houses in which they live are subsidized by the LAs either directly or through housing associations. People with mental handicaps are supported by social workers, home helps, and others, sometimes including members of their family, as necessary. Many are not truly independent. Some of the people who live independently are capable of sustained employment, sometimes in sheltered workshops, but may have difficulties in areas of high unemployment.

NHS hostels

A few hostels have been built to accommodate people who have been displaced from the old-style mental handicap hospitals. Some of these hostels have been built on the same campuses as the mental handicap hospitals, and are used as half-way houses; others are specifically designed for people with a high degree of dependency. There are also a small number of ordinary residential houses managed by the NHS authorities. Of the people on the registers, 82 (1.4%) currently live in NHS hostels.

Group homes

The term 'group home' is an ill-defined term used to describe houses in the community that may be run by social services, voluntary organizations, or the NHS. There are 156 people (2.7%) described as living in such accommodation.

Other

This category includes people living in old people's homes, part III accommodation, church army hostels, residences for the physically handicapped, or other types of establishment (see below).

There are striking differences in the ages of people in different types of accommodation. Figure 4.1 shows the proportion of individuals in each age group who are resident in the four types of residence that are used most frequently. The proportion living in their family homes decreases with increasing age; the proportion living in hospital increases with age; beyond the age of 15, the proportion living in P/V accommodation remains relatively constant; up to the age of 15, nearly 90% reside in the family home, and there are very few in hospital.

Although the proportion of those over age 65 who are in hospital is high, the overall numbers of people in this age group in hospital is small (Figure 4.2). An issue of great interest

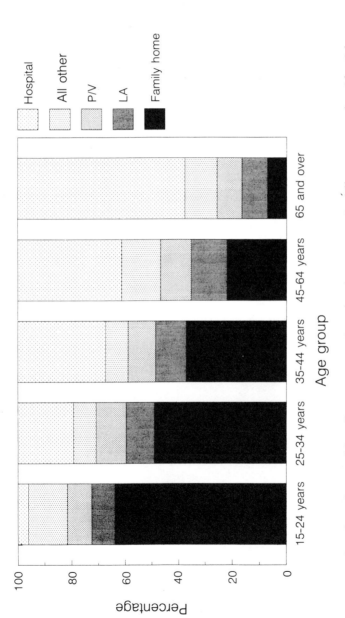

Figure 4.1 People with mental handicaps – proportion of each age group in different types of residential accommodation.

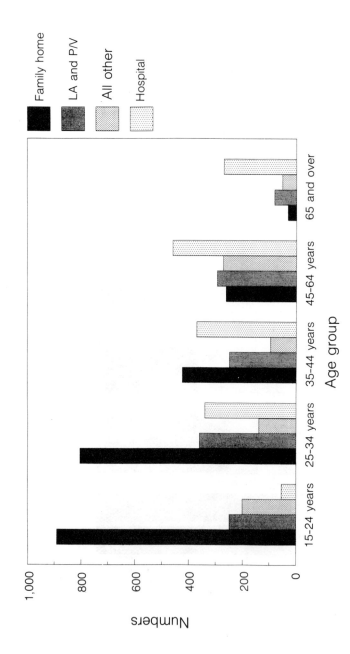

Figure 4.2 People with mental handicaps – numbers in each age group in different types of residential accommodation.

is the numbers of adults in the younger age groups who are living with their families; there are about 2100 such people between the ages of 15–44. The available evidence indicates that there are virtually no free places in private and voluntary homes, local authority, or NHS homes, or in any other type of specialized accommodation. This, coupled with the policy of closing hospitals to new admissions, indicates that there may well be a crisis in the future, when many of those now living in the family home will no longer be able to do so as a result of death or illness of the principal carer. A major change in approach to residential care and significant capital and revenue investment clearly will be required within the next decade.

There is considerable variation between districts in the way in which different types of residence are used (Table 4.1). The proportion registered as living at home with their family varies between 28.8% in KCW and 67.7% in North Hertfordshire. North Hertfordshire has the lowest proportion in hospital (7.4%), and Hammersmith and Fulham has the highest (34.6%).

KCW and Harrow make extensive use of the P/V sector; KCW uses very little LA accommodation. Some of these differences may be due to inconsistencies in the rate of registration between different residential settings; for example, the remarkably low percentage in hospital from North Hertfordshire, coupled with their low overall numbers suggests that relatively few of their hospital cases are registered – rather

Table 4.1 Percentages in different types of residential accommodation

	Home	Hospital	LA hostel	P/V home	Other
Brent	44.1	24.0	7.3	9.0	15.6
E. Herts	54.1	17.5	8.1	5.4	14.8
H'Smith	29.5	34.6	6.0	15.0	14.7
Harrow	37.6	27.5	14.3	13.1	7.5
Hill'don	58.3	15.9	18.1	0.5	6.8
H. and S.	53.7	32.6	5.3	3.4	5.1
N. Herts	67.7	7.4	7.1	4.1	13.8
S. Beds	51.4	20.7	14.2	5.9	7.8
S.W. Herts	41.8	27.3	10.4	10.0	10.5
KCW	28.8	24.9	4.8	27.1	14.4

than that most of those for whom they are responsible have left hospital. However, there remains a significant interdistrict variation in the use of LA compared with P/V hostel accommodation, and in the proportions living in the family home.

In subsequent chapters the characteristics of people living in their family homes, of the residents of hospitals, in P/V homes, in LA homes and hostels, and people in other types of residence will be discussed in detail.

5

Residents in family homes

Age distribution

The average age of people over 15 years with mental handicaps who live in the family home is 30.06 years (SD 11.56). They are younger than those resident in institutions or other types of accommodation (average age 42.05; SD 16.70). Figure 5.1 compares the age distribution of people who live with their families with all other people with mental handicaps. More than 90% of those living at home are under age 45, whereas 64% of those living in places other than the family home are under the age of 45. This is not surprising, as the availability of a family home is normally dependent upon the survival and health of at least one of the parents, usually the mother.

In 'normal' populations, children tend to leave home and establish independent lives in their late 'teens and early 20s. The fact that a high proportion of those who have handicaps and who are still living with their families are over 30 is of importance. With increasing age of the handicapped person, the probability of survival of the key parent decreases. The use of the family home by a person with mental handicap is thus inevitably time limited.

The present situation has arisen first because hospitals have effectively been closed to admissions for some years, in particular for children. Even if parents wished their offspring to be cared for in such institutions, provision has not been available. Second, to a great extent the new places created in

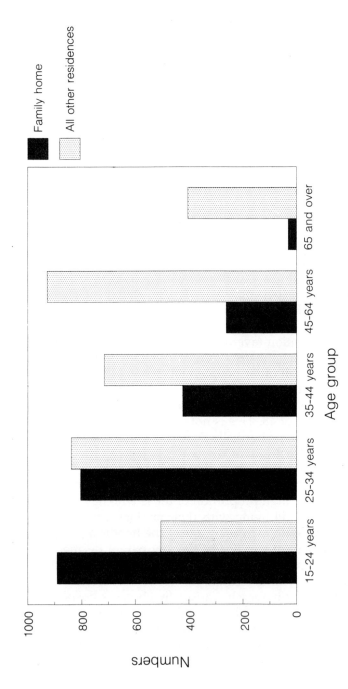

Figure 5.1 People with mental handicaps – numbers in each age group in family homes compared with all others.

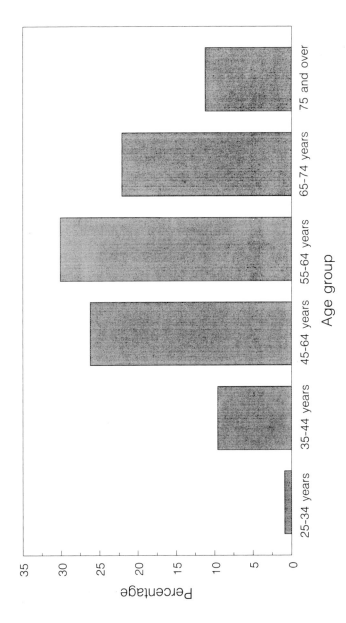

Figure 5.2 Main carer – proportion in each age group.

the 'community' have been provided for and taken by people discharged from hospitals, rather than having been made available for people who, in previous years, would have been admitted to hospital. This suggests that in the future a crisis will occur as the principal carers of people with mental handicaps die, or otherwise become unable to provide the necessary care and support.

Age of principal carer

The distribution of people resident in their family homes according to the age of their principal carer (where known) is shown in Figure 5.2. In planning terms, it could be argued that the age of the principal carer is more important than the age of the person with a mental handicap.

Nearly half of the carers are now over the age of 60 years. It is possible to forecast the likely numbers of people with mental handicaps who will lose their principal carer in successive years, if it is assumed that the life expectancy of people who care for a mentally handicapped family member is the same as that of the general population. By 1994, 238 of the 2412 carers – about 10% – can be expected to have died. By 1999, this number will have risen to 512. There will be no real alternative to the 'children' of these people being taken into residential care of some type.

Many believe people should be able to leave home either when they want to, or when their parents either want or need them to. Using death as the only end-point of care in the family home grossly under-estimates the scale of provision of residential accommodation likely to be required in the foreseeable future.

If the principle is accepted that, except in special circumstances, all people over the age of 25 should live away from their parents – this being the norm for those who are not mentally handicapped – then the number of residential places that will be required over the next decade will be dependent on the ages of the mentally handicapped people who are now living at home and at boarding school. There are 2481 people over 15 years living at home – in ten years' time all should have been offered the option of leaving home.

The current situation is further complicated by the fact that the numbers of people with mental handicaps born in the 1960s – now aged 20–29 years – appears to be greater than in the past, as a result of the second post-war birth bulge, and increased survival from vulnerable pregnancies.

In the 1960s there was an increase in the numbers of births because of the relatively high numbers of women in the UK who attained childbearing age. These women were born towards the end of, and just after, the Second World War, when there was a net increase in birth rate. At the same time, the technology for the management of premature and abnormal labour, and some of the previously unmanageable conditions of the foetus – for example, rhesus incompatibility – was greatly improved. Although these developments resulted in a reduction in perinatal mortality, a higher proportion of these babies compared with normal pregnancies were handi-capped from birth.

Fryers (1984) discussed possible additional causes for the increase in numbers of people with mental handicaps born in the late 1960s at some length. He postulated that it might include:

- Better case-finding, creating an apparent bulge when in fact those born earlier were simply not recorded, and may subsequently have died.
- Stability of families with a handicapped member, where the rest of the population may be leaving the area; or, alternatively, differential migration into areas with better services.
- Life-saving antibiotic treatment for chest infections, a major problem for those with Down's syndrome, who form the biggest diagnostic group within the larger group of mentally handicapped people.
- The increase in family, as opposed to institutional care for handicapped children.

Parsons (1963) and Miller *et al.* (1987) have argued that immi-grant mothers are susceptible to rubella infection, not having been exposed to the infection in their country of birth, and having therefore acquired no natural immunity, and there being no immunization offered on arrival in this country. Both have recorded a higher than expected incidence of congenital rubella in immigrant populations, of which those from the West Indies and southern Asia (India, Pakistan, Bangladesh, and Sri Lanka) have the greatest excess.

Although in most cases the principal carer is the mother, for a few people the principal carer and next-of-kin are of the same generation – a brother or sister. This is particularly true of the elderly. It is necessary to consider the long-term viability of a system of care which is partly dependent upon siblings taking on the long-term responsibility for their middle-aged relatives with mental handicaps. Although this arrangement might provide a short-term solution while there is inadequate special accommodation, it should be a matter of choice by all concerned rather than forced by circumstances.

Day activities

Most of those who lived at home were involved with some type of activity during the day. The younger individuals attended special schools, most of which were day schools. Only a small proportion attended boarding school. Clearly, attendance at day school places greater demands on the family than having a child at a boarding school. Parents may choose day school places because they prefer to have their child at home with them, or the choice may be a forced one because of a lack of acceptable boarding places.

After school age, the majority of people with mental handicaps who lived in their family home and were under 65 years old attended social and education centres (SECs) or equivalents (adult training centres (ATCs), day centres, and so on). Many of these centres provide facilities for several hours a day, and most are open throughout the year. However, most of the centres are full, have long waiting lists, and are reluctant to accept people with challenging behaviours. The reduction in the number of mental handicap hospital places is causing additional pressure.

44

Table 5.1 Principal day-time activities of those in the family home in each age group (%)

	Age group		
	15–29	*30–44*	*>45*
None	3.7	10.6	19.5
Day school	36.5	0.0	0.0
Boarding school	0.9	0.0	0.0
Home teaching	0.2	0.0	0.0
College	3.5	0.5	0.7
Work experience	0.6	0.3	0.0
ATC/SEC	42.6	70.9	53.6
Sheltered employment	0.5	0.5	0.7
Open employment	1.2	4.3	4.4
Other	1.9	2.5	3.4
NK	8.4	10.5	17.7
Total individuals	1440	748	293

More places are urgently needed in day provision for those about to leave school and those being resettled from the hospitals. It is unlikely that a substantial number of places will be vacated in the next ten years within the SECs because most of the current users are young. It follows that consideration should be given to an expansion of capital and manpower investment in this sector if the hospital closure programme is to continue at its present pace.

Very few people with mental handicaps who lived at home were employed (3.1%), either in sheltered workshops or elsewhere. It is possible, although unlikely, that this was partly related to the general level of unemployment; the most likely explanation is that their disabilities and handicaps were incompatible with the type of employment available.

The day-time activities of those who lived in their family home is shown in Table 5.1. In the 15–29 age group, the majority were either at school or attended an ATC or SEC. The ATCs and SECs were the most important day-time activities among those over 30 years of age.

Only an insignificant percentage of the people with mental handicaps who lived in the family home are employed, either in sheltered or open jobs. In this respect, many of the hopes and expectations expressed by successive committees that people with mental handicaps would be employed have not been fulfilled. In fact, only 8.5% of all those who lived at home did anything other than attend special schools, 'training' centres, or SECs – all of which are specifically and exclusively provided for people with mental handicaps.

Degree of mental handicap

The degree of mental handicap of those who were living in the family home is shown in Table 5.2. The category 'Using Mental Handicap Services' does not form part of the International Classification of Diseases (ICD). It is used here to designate those who did not fit into the standard categories available, as they were deemed to have an IQ of over 70. The category ICD 319 (Unspecified Mental Retardation), is used either because the assessor did not know, or because the assessor was unwilling to classify the individual. The 'Not Known' (NK) category is used for cases where no information was available on the registers. There was no information on the degree of mental handicap in over half of the cases. Of those who were assigned to a discrete category, 49.5% were deemed to be either severely or profoundly mentally handicapped.

Table 5.2 Degree of mental handicap of people living in family home

		Age group				
		15–29	*30–44*	*45–64*	*⩾65*	*All*
Using mental handicap services		32	27	9	1	69
ICD code						
317	Mild mental retardation	174	149	54	5	381
318.0	Moderate mental retardation	218	125	31	1	375
318.1	Severe mental retardation	324	72	18	0	414
318.2	Profound mental retardation	52	10	3	0	65
319	Unspecified mental retardation	466	244	95	15	820
	NK	159	112	51	8	330
Total		1440	748	262	31	2481

Abilities and disabilities

Continence

Four different assessments of continence were made: night and day urinary incontinence, and night and day faecal incontinence. Each was assessed on a three-point scale: frequent (more than once per week), occasionally, and never. The distribution of those who lived at home over the age of 15 years according to these categories is shown in Table 5.3.

Between 6–12% of all those who lived in the family home frequently have some form of incontinence (Table 5.3). Clearly, some people fell into the 'Frequent' or 'Severe' category for more than one of the indices of incontinence. Table 5.4 shows the percentages of people in each age group who had any form of incontinence.

Table 5.3 Assessment of continence – residents in family home > 15 years. ( ) = percentages of those known

	NK	Frequent	Occasional	Never
Urinary/day	333	172 (10.4)	224 (8.0)	1752 (81.6)
Urinary/night	386	257 (13.0)	273 (12.3)	1565 (74.7)
Faecal/day	335	136 (8.7)	186 (6.3)	1824 (85.0)
Faecal/night	392	140 (7.4)	154 (6.7)	1795 (85.9)

Table 5.4 People living in family homes who have at least one problem of incontinence – rated either 'frequently' or 'occasionally' – as a percentage of all in that age group

	Cases	Incontinent	% Incontinent
15–29	1251	468	37.4
30–44	641	110	17.2
45–64	223	32	14.3
65 +	21	5	23.8
All	2136	615	28.8

The percentage of people with some form of incontinence decreased with increasing age. This might have been the result of selective admission to institutional care, or because the younger cohorts were not admitted to institutions in the same numbers as the older groups. It is unlikely that the trends with age were the result of continence being established after the age of 30. Irrespective of the explanation for the trend with age, the fact remains that the relatives of about 29% of the people with mental handicaps who lived at home had to cope with incontinence.

Mobility

Of those living in their family home, 86.8% were able to walk by themselves and climb stairs. Although they were rated as mobile, many had some degree of spasticity or other problems of co-ordination; 6.5% could not manage to climb stairs without assistance, 6.8% could not walk at all.

Of those who could not walk unaided, 70% were unable to do so even with assistance from another person; 8.2% of the total group had a wheelchair; only about one in seven of these were able to manage their chair on their own.

Sensory function, communication, and literacy

Seven measures of sensory function, communication, and literacy were included in the assessment: sight; hearing; speech; understanding; reading ability; writing ability; and counting ability.

Of all those who were resident in the family home, 2.3% were blind, and a further 17.2% had very poor vision; 1.7% were deaf, and 7.1% had poor hearing; 3.9% had a combination of visual and auditory handicaps; 0.3% were both blind and deaf.

Those who had no speech totalled 13.5%, and a further 13.5% were only able to ask for their basic needs; 3.5% were rated as having no ability to understand either speech or gesture; 14.0% were only able to understand basic communication through speech or gesture.

Not surprisingly, only 20% could read at all, and 19% were able to count enough to be able to manage small amounts of money; 14% were able to write their own correspondence.

Self-help skills

Apart from the problems of incontinence and mobility, the lack of ability of some people with mental handicaps to look after themselves in the most basic ways places additional demands on the family. Among these are the ability to wash, dress, and feed themselves. Table 5.5 shows the percentages who had problems in this area.

Over 40% of the people with mental handicaps who were being cared for by their families needed help with washing; just under 40% required assistance with dressing; and 15% could not feed themselves without some help. These disabilities were likely to entail a full-time commitment of at least one member of the family (Dupont, 1980), and create difficulties when the key carer wishes to have a holiday or relax outside the home.

Table 5.5 Personal living skills of individuals living in the family home (percentages)

Skill	NK	Not at all	With help	Without help	All with assessment
Feed self	298	104 (4.8)	220 (10.1)	1859 (85.2)	2183 (100)
Wash self	308	272 (12.5)	636 (29.3)	1265 (58.2)	2173 (100)
Dress self	311	219 (10.1)	574 (26)	1377 (63.5)	2170 (100)

Problems with behaviour

It is important to know about the person's behaviour for two principal reasons. First, people with mental handicaps often have difficulties with speech or signing communications, and their behaviour may reflect their pain, anxiety, loneliness, unhappiness, boredom, and frustration. Second, an appreciation of the behavioural difficulties of individuals is necessary in order to plan for appropriate placements and interventions.

Its significance cannot be ignored. Ten types of behaviour were assessed and classified, as follows:

1. Often a severe problem.
2. Occasionally a severe problem.
3. Often a mild problem.
4. Occasionally a mild problem.
5. Never a problem.

The percentage distribution of the cases over 15 years of age for whom data were available according to their rating of each of the behaviours is shown in Table 5.6. Categories one and two have been amalgamated to form the category 'Severe'; categories three and four are amalgamated to form the category 'Mild'.

Table 5.6 Behavioural problems according to severity (percentages)

Behaviour	Severe	Mild	None
Attention-seeking	8.6	22.0	69.4
Damaging property	4.7	11.1	84.2
Delinquent acts	1.7	4.4	93.9
Noise	8.3	19.8	71.9
Over-active	7.2	15.8	77.0
Objectionable personal habits	2.4	7.4	90.2
Personal aggression	5.6	17.0	77.4
Self-injury	4.8	11.6	83.6
Wandering off	4.3	11.8	83.9
Withdrawn	8.0	26.3	65.7

The most frequently encountered 'Severe' problems were attention-seeking (8.6%); noise (8.3%); over-activity (7.2%); and being withdrawn (8.0%). Although 'attention-seeking' and 'withdrawal' might be thought to be mutually exclusive, this is not the case; some people exhibited both behaviours at different times – it is likely that the combination of the two made caring more difficult.

The term 'delinquent acts' covers most of the types of behaviour that may result in the involvement of the police, for example, shoplifting, fire-raising, indecent exposure. Relatively few of those resident in their family homes created such problems, but when they do occur it causes great distress to all involved. A small percentage have 'objectionable personal habits', for example, spitting, faecal smearing, and so on. Although rare, they are distressing when they do occur. A higher proportion showed 'personal aggression', for example, hitting or kicking other people, often for no apparent reason.

Table 5.7 shows the frequency of 'Severe' problems in different age groups. In all behaviours the frequency decreases with increasing age. It is likely this was because people who had severe behavioural problems were selectively admitted to institutional care as they, or their carers, aged.

Table 5.7 Percentage with severe behavioural problems (often or occasional) by age group (residents in family home only)

| | Age group | | | | |
Behaviour	15–29	30–44	45–64	65+	All > 15
Attention-seeking	10.9	5.8	4.2	0.0	8.6
Damaging property	6.9	2.0	0.9	0.0	4.7
Delinquent acts	2.3	1.0	0.5	0.0	1.7
Noise	11.1	4.3	3.8	(5.2)*	8.3
Over-active	9.8	3.8	1.9	(9.5)*	7.2
Objectionable personal habits	3.5	1.0	0.0	0.0	2.4
Personal aggression	7.1	3.6	2.8	0.0	5.6
Self-injury	7.0	2.0	0.5	4.8	4.8
Wandering off	6.2	1.7	1.4	0.0	4.3
Withdrawn	9.8	6.1	3.8	4.8	8.0

*( ) less than 3 cases

Combinations of disabilities and problems

Thus far, each disability or problem has been considered separately. There were, however, many people with mental handicaps who had multiple problems and disabilities. In order to assess the importance of these, 'Severe Physical Score' and a 'Severe Behavioural Score' has been assigned to each individual. This score was generated by counting the number of 'Severe' ratings for each of the 12 physical and 10 behavioural parameters. People with scores of 0 had no 'Severe' problems on either axis, however they may have had problems rated other than as severe in either axis. In short, this method is designed to identify only the most severely disabled.

Table 5.8 shows the distribution of cases according to their 'Severe Physical' and 'Severe Behavioural' scores: 64.3% did not have any 'Severe' behavioural or physical problems; the remainder (35.8%) had at least one severe problem recorded. As the physical score increases, the proportion with high behavioural scores tends to decrease. Conversely, as the behavioural score increases, the proportion with high physical scores decreases. This is not surprising, as the greater the physical handicap the less is the scope for behavioural problems. There were, however, a number of people with high physical and behavioural scores. Clearly these individuals would have needed constant and intensive care.

Table 5.8 Distribution of 'Severe Physical' and 'Severe Behavioural' problems amongst people living in their family homes aged > 15 years

Number of severe physical problems	Number of severe behavioural problems				
	0	1–2	3–5	>5	Total
0	1594	182	63	13	1852
1–2	254	74	34	12	374
3–5	62	31	17	7	117
>5	91	34	12	1	138
Total	2001	321	126	33	2481

Illustrative cases

The problems of some of the people resident in their family homes were at least as great as those resident in hospital. This can be illustrated by the following examples of individual cases.

Case A was a 33-year-old profoundly handicapped woman who lived at home and was cared for by her 65-year-old mother. She had tuberous sclerosis, pyschotic symptoms, and her epilepsy was only partially controlled. She was frequently doubly incontinent at night, and occasionally so during the day. She was fully mobile and could feed herself, but could neither wash nor dress herself. She had only basic speech and understanding. She had severe behavioural problems, including being aggressive to people, and was prone to damage property, and to be overactive. She attended a special unit at the local SEC during weekdays.

Case B was a 17-year-old severely mentally handicapped boy with partially controlled epilepsy cared for by his 44-year-old mother. He was doubly incontinent. He was mobile but needed help with feeding, and could not wash or dress himself at all. He had no speech and no signing communication, but was reported to have basic understanding. He had a number of severe behaviour problems, including wandering off, aggression to people, and objectionable personal habits. He attended a day school during the week.

Case C was a 20-year-old severely mentally handicapped man with controlled epilepsy. He was cared for by his 52-year-old mother. He was doubly incontinent. He could not walk on his own, and could not manage his wheelchair without help. He needed help with feeding, and could not wash or dress himself at all. He had no speech and no understanding. His personal habits were a problem. He attended a day school.

Case D was a 25-year-old woman with Down's syndrome who was looked after by her 52-year-old mother. She was doubly incontinent, could not wash or dress herself at all, and had no speech. She had only basic understanding. She was withdrawn, and tended to injure herself. She attended an ATC.

These cases should not be regarded as typical, since each individual has his or her unique combination of disabilities, and presents different problems for the carers. Most are totally dependent upon their mother. These cases are highlighted because the received wisdom is that people now living in the family home are less disabled than those in institutional care; the evidence is that this was not the case. Continued residence at home for people with multiple disabilities can, at best, only be regarded as a temporary arrangement.

Comparison of people living in family homes with residents in other places

In order to establish the principal characteristics that distinguish them, the proportion in the family home group who were positive for each of the indices was compared with the proportion positive in all other types of residential accommodation. There were statistically significant differences at the 1% level on 16 of the indices (Table 5.9).

People with mental handicaps who reside at home were found to be more likely to have problems with vision, feeding, and over-activity than those living elsewhere. They were less likely to have problems with night urinary incontinence; night

Table 5.9 Distribution of each of the variables for people living in the family home compared with all other people with mental handicaps (significant at P < 01)

Variable	Chi^2	Prob	Direction
Urinary incontinence/night	13.98	0.001	Less
Faecal incontinence/night	12.61	0.002	Less
Urinary incontinence/day	14.13	0.001	Less
Faecal incontinence/day	6.12	NS	
Walking	23.73	0.000	Less
Feeding	26.30	0.000	More
Washing	8.19	NS	
Dressing	8.73	NS	
Vision	33.08	0.000	More
Hearing	12.59	0.002	Less
Speech	64.43	0.000	Less
Understanding	32.96	0.000	Less
Personal aggression	70.53	0.000	Less
Damaging	27.54	0.000	Less
Over-active	13.65	0.008	More
Attention-seeking	7.81	NS	
Self-injury	16.25	0.003	Less
Delinquent	129.63	0.000	Less
Personal habits	120.82	0.000	Less
Wandering	4.58	NS	
Noise	37.34	0.000	Less
Withdrawn	22.26	0.000	Less

Less = Fewer severe problems among people living in the family home than all others on the registers.
More = More severe problems among people living in their family home than all others on the registers.

faecal incontinence; daytime urinary incontinence; mobility; hearing; speech; understanding; personal aggression; damaging property; self-injury; unpleasant personal habits; delinquent behaviour; being withdrawn; and being noisy. There was no significant difference in the frequency of the other indices measured.

Summary

People with mental handicaps who lived in their own homes had a comparatively high incidence of disabilities: 29% were incontinent; 13% had substantial mobility problems; 20% had visual problems; and nearly 9% had hearing problems; 27% had only basic speech or could not speak at all; 40% needed help most of the time with feeding, washing, and dressing. In addition, nearly 36% had at least one behavioural problem.

A substantial percentage of them had problems that devolved not only around needs such as washing, dressing, feeding, and toileting, but included physical and behavioural problems of considerable severity.

The average age of people over 15 years who lived in their family homes was about 30 years, and over 45% of their carers were over the age of 60 years.

They remained at home because of a combination of five factors:

- Places in the community were mostly taken by people who had been discharged from hospitals.
- Hospital admission was difficult or impossible because of current policies.
- Residential provision that was available outside hospital was often unsuitable for those who were dependent and multiply handicapped.
- Sometimes parents found the alternative accommodation unacceptable.
- Some parents wished to continue to care for their handicapped 'child'.

Few in this group would be able to live independently. Some of them are unlikely to be accepted by any of the current non-hospital residential facilities. Their 'total disability score' as a group was second only to that of the hospital residents, and the fact that a high percentage of them had aged parents – a significant proportion of whom are likely to die each year – gives rise to concern. It is estimated that about 50 people will have to be re-housed each year because of the death of the relative who provided care. At present there appear to be no concrete plans or finance to meet this definable need.

6

Residents in hospitals

Introduction

In the UK, until the mid-1970s most of the residential care for people with mental handicaps was provided in hospitals, which still provide about 23% of all the accommodation for this group. Although many of the hospitals are geographically isolated, and are now forbidding, antiquated in design, and poorly maintained, when they were built they represented the best and most generous of provision. Their construction was the result of a minor social revolution: for the first time it was recognized that people with mental handicaps required special facilities, and that their families were entitled to be relieved of a lifetime burden of care.

Initially, and for many years after the opening of the public hospitals for people with mental handicaps, the practice was to 'certify' affected individuals in order to admit them. One of the reasons for 'certification' was that the residential places were so desirable, and a method was needed of ensuring that only those people for whom they were designed were admitted.

Few of those 'certified' and admitted ever returned to the community from which they originated. Sometimes mistakes were made in the assessment of individuals; sometimes the system was frankly abused – for example, there are documented examples of young women having been certified as moral defectives and detained in hospital for the remainder of their lives because they had become pregnant out of wedlock.

Since the mid-1970s, there has been an explicit policy of discharging people from hospitals with a view to 'resettling' them in the communities from which they came, and then closing the hospitals. This policy was not unique to the UK, and has been attempted in other European countries, the US, and Canada. The new policy of the 1970s was coupled with a rigorous selection procedure for admission, or re-admission.

The current hospital population comprises two more or less distinct groups: those who were admitted when institutional care was the accepted norm; and those who have been admitted since the mid-1970s.

Provision in NW Thames

The age distribution of those who lived in hospital is different from that of people who lived in their own family homes (Figure 6.1). Of hospital residents, 18.1% are aged over 65 years compared with 1.3% of the people who live in their family homes.

Figure 6.2 shows the numbers of hospital residents according to the year of their admission to the hospital in which they were resident; some might have been resident in other hospitals before. The people who were admitted earliest first entered hospital between 1918–20. Thus, some had been in hospital continuously for 70 years. The number in each admission cohort would have been reduced by death and by the implementation of recent discharge policies. There is no way of establishing how many were admitted each year in the early part of this century. It is likely that the numbers who were admitted before the 1950s would have been reduced mainly by death, and the numbers who were admitted subsequently would have been reduced by resettlement. However, there does appear to have been a sharp fall in the numbers admitted after the mid-1970s.

The average age at admission of hospital residents according to their year of admission is shown in Figure 6.3.

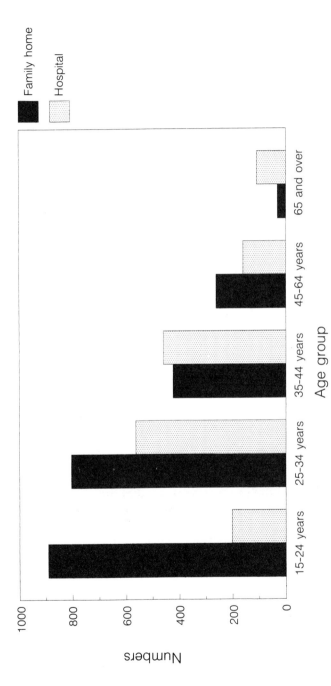

Figure 6.1 People with mental handicaps – numbers in each age group in family home compared with all in hospital.

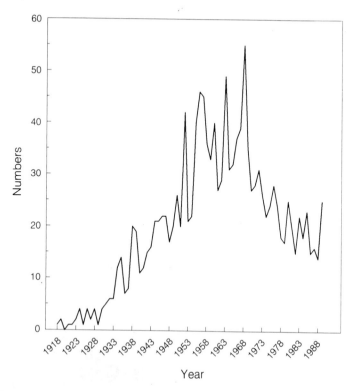

Figure 6.2 NW Thames RHA – people with mental handicaps (hospital residents by year of admission).

The reasons for the low average ages at admission of people first admitted in the pre-war period is that the older residents would have died. Therefore, these data cannot be used to investigate the long-term trends in age at admission. Nevertheless, it is possible to identify a striking recent change. The average age at admission increased by 10 to 15 years between 1971 and 1972. This sudden change was unlikely to have been due to differences in survival; it was more likely to have been a reflection of a change in admissions policy.

There are four major mental handicap hospitals within the NW Thames Region: Leavesden, Bromham, Cell Barnes, and Harperbury. None of them are used exclusively by districts

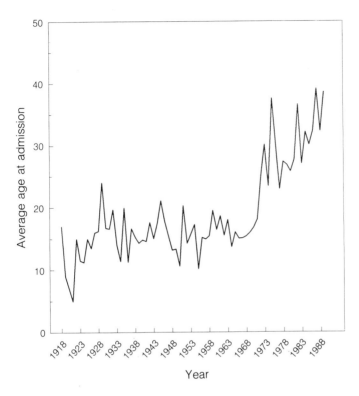

Figure 6.3 NW Thames RHA – people with mental handicaps living in hospital (average age at admission by year of admission).

within the region. Some districts use other hospitals outside the regional boundaries. Table 6.1 shows the numbers of persons with mental handicaps included on the registers who were resident in different hospitals. Nearly 70% of all the NW Thames hospital cases registered were resident in hospitals managed by the districts in the NW Thames region.

The age distribution of people on the registers who were resident in the main hospitals is shown in Table 6.2. There were substantial differences between hospitals. The Bromham, St Ebba's, Kingsbury, and Normansfield residents comprised the youngest group. The Harperbury, Manor, and Fairfield residents were the oldest. The variations in age distribution

Residents in hospitals

Table 6.1 People with mental handicaps originating from the NW Thames RHA now resident in hospitals

Hospital	Cases	% of all hospital cases
Hospitals in NW Thames region		
Leavesden	316	21.2
Cell Barnes	232	15.5
Bromham	226	15.1
Harperbury	218	14.6
Kingsbury	51	3.4
Subtotal	1043	69.8
Hospitals outside NW Thames region		
St Lawrence's	104	7.0
Manor	57	3.8
St Ebbas's	50	3.3
Fairfield	42	2.8
Normansfield	37	2.5
Other hospitals	161	10.8
Total	1494	100.0

Table 6.2 Ages of residents in the main hospitals used – percentages in each age group, mean age and standard deviation

Hospital	15–29	30–44	45–64	65+	Mean age	SD
Leavesden	18.6	37.7	24.7	19.0	46.39	17.22
Cell Barnes	13.4	40.1	33.6	12.9	45.50	14.51
Bromham	23.5	42.0	18.1	9.5	40.80	15.10
Harperbury	0.0	27.5	44.5	27.1	54.74	14.46
Kingsbury	21.6	39.2	29.4	9.8	42.90	15.60
St Lawrence's	0.0	31.7	48.1	19.2	53.19	13.28
Manor	5.3	19.3	28.1	47.4	59.09	15.81
St Ebbas's	0.0	72.0	26.0	2.0	42.06	7.50
Fairfield	2.4	4.8	38.1	54.8	65.00	13.34
Normansfield	10.8	54.1	27.0	8.1	43.00	12.49

reflect changes in catchment areas and admission policies over the past 50 years, together with recent differences in resettlement policy.

The numbers presented here are **not** the total numbers in hospital from the NW Thames Region – it has already been established that the database is incomplete in some districts, and that two districts are missing altogether. The findings from the districts with reliable data can be extrapolated to the regional population as a whole. Thus there were at least 2240 people from the NW Thames region resident in hospital. If the hospitals are to be closed within the next decade, about two-thirds of these people (1500) will have to be resettled – the remainder are unlikely to survive the decade.

Day-time activity
Although a range of educational, training, and work activities were provided in the hospitals, a considerable proportion of residents in each age group were not involved in any of them (Table 6.3). There was considerable variation between hospitals. School and skills development workshops were the principal activities of the younger residents, whereas occupational therapy was the main activity of those who were older.

Table 6.3 Principal day activities of those living in hospital – percentages in each age group

	Age group		
Activity	*15–29*	*30–44*	*> 45*
None	30.8	29.9	39.2
School	20.0	4.6	0.9
Skills development unit	17.8	13.1	9.2
Industrial workshop	3.0	6.8	5.2
Farm unit	0.0	0.2	0.5
Garden unit	0.4	1.3	0.5
Occupational therapy	7.4	16.2	18.0
Behaviour modification	6.5	6.3	0.8
Working in hospital	0.9	3.2	11.5
Open employment	0.4	0.2	0.4
Other	11.3	16.7	11.1
NK	0.9	1.6	2.8

Table 6.4 Principal day activities of those living in hospital – percentages in different length-of-stay categories

	Length of stay (years)			
Activity	1–2	3–5	6–15	> 15
None	51.6	28.8	22.2	35.9
School	6.5	13.7	4.9	4.3
Skills development unit	6.5	9.6	18.4	10.4
Industrial workshop	0.0	5.5	6.9	5.4
Farm unit	0.0	0.0	0.3	0.4
Garden unit	6.5	2.7	1.4	0.4
Occupational therapy	12.9	12.3	22.2	15.0
Behaviour modification	0.0	5.5	4.5	1.8
Working in hospital	3.2	0.0	4.5	9.9
Open employment	3.2	1.4	0.3	0.2
Other	6.5	2.7	13.2	14.0
NK	3.2	4.1	1.0	2.2

Very few were involved in the 'traditional' activities of the long-stay hospitals – farming and gardening – which some regarded as being both enjoyable and rewarding.

The age of residents in hospital was generally closely related to their duration of stay, however, the differences in the day-time activities of residents according to length of stay revealed an interesting phenomenon: the majority, who had been resident for under three years, were not involved in any formal day-time activity; the schools, skills development units, and occupational therapy units were used mostly by the long-established residents (Table 6.4). This may have been because the more recently admitted patients were more likely to be behaviourally disturbed and difficult to involve in any organized activity, or it could have been due to difficulties in making arrangements for those who were inpatients for short periods. It might also have been related to a net deficit of resources within the institutions.

Degree of mental handicap

Table 6.5 shows the numbers in hospital by age and degree of handicap. A higher proportion of hospital patients were

Table 6.5 Degree of mental handicap of people living in hospital

ICD code		Age group				
		15–29	30–44	45–64	≥65	All
	Using MH services.	6	31	30	15	82
317	Mild mental retard.	11	59	68	71	209
318.0	Mod. mental retard.	19	86	110	79	294
318.1	Sev. mental retard.	111	298	187	86	682
318.2	Prof. mental retard	39	62	39	6	146
319	Unspec. mental retard.	16	25	24	12	77
	NK	0	2	1	1	4
Total		202	563	459	270	1494

'Severely' or 'Profoundly' handicapped than those who were living in their family home. This was due in part to the selective resettlement of those who were less disabled (Farmer *et al.*, 1990), and in part to selective admission policies. As the resettlement policy continues, it is to be expected that the proportion of the residual hospital population who are either profoundly or severely handicapped will increase.

Among those whose degree of mental handicap was known, 21.7% in the age group 15–29 were profoundly handicapped. The proportion who were profoundly handicapped decreased with age: 12.3% aged 30–44 years; 9.7% aged 45–64 years; and 2.5% aged 65 years and over. This striking decrease in the proportion so handicapped was likely to be due to differential survival and changes in admission and resettlement policy. The present generation of profoundly handicapped people are likely to survive longer than those from earlier birth cohorts, which has important implications for future service provision.

Abilities and disabilities

Continence of hospital patients was recorded in the same way as for people living in their own family homes. Details were available on a greater proportion of the hospital patients than for home residents. The prevalence and frequency of all four types of incontinence was higher than among people at home (Table 6.6). Only 54.4% of people living in hospital were fully continent, compared to 74.7% of those in the family home.

The proportion in each age and duration-of-stay group who had a 'frequent' problem of either urinary or faecal incontinence either during the day or during the night is shown in Table 6.7. There is a general, although weak, trend for the proportion of residents affected to decrease with age and increase with duration of stay. It is likely that the most severely affected were admitted at a younger age, and the less severe had already been resettled in the community.

Mobility – 67.1% of those living in hospital were both able to walk by themselves and climb stairs, a smaller percentage than among those living in their family homes (86.8%). In both

Table 6.6 Continence – residents in hospital aged > 15 years, ( ) = percent of known

	NK	Frequent	Occasional	Never
Urinary/day	21	276 (18.7)	312 (21.2)	885 (60.1)
Urinary/night	21	338 (22.9)	334 (22.7)	801 (54.4)
Faecal/day	21	195 (13.2)	286 (19.4)	992 (67.3)
Faecal/night	21	212 (14.4)	276 (18.7)	984 (66.8)

Table 6.7 Hospital residents with at least one problem of 'frequent' incontinence according to age now and duration of stay in hospital (percentage)

Duration of stay years	Age group			
	15–29	30–44	45–64	> 64
0–9	50.6	29.4	37.5	25.0
10–19	72.7	50.0	41.8	48.6
20–29		58.1	28.4	41.4
30–39		62.2	47.5	37.8
40–49			51.8	47.4
50–59			41.9	40.8

environments, even those who were rated as fully mobile may have had a considerable degree of spasticity or other physical difficulties, which made their progress slow or painful: 17.6% could not manage stairs, and a further 17.6% were unable to walk without help. Eight out of ten of the latter could not walk, even with help. Of all the people in hospital, 17.9% had wheelchairs, less than one-quarter of whom were able to manage the chairs on their own.

The younger hospital residents had a higher prevalence of mobility problems (Table 6.8). In order to establish whether or not this phenomenon was due to changes in admission criteria, the mobility assessments were analysed by admission year. There is no indication of an association. It is difficult to explain the higher prevalence of problems of mobility among the younger residents, other than that there seems to be a differential survival between the severely and less-severely physically disabled (Eyman, 1990).

Table 6.8 Hospital residents with mobility problems according to age group (percentages)

Ability to walk	Age group			
	15–29	30–44	45–64	>64
NK	0.5	2.5	1.4	0.6
Not at all	22.8	16.9	10.5	13.3
With help	7.4	13.9	19.4	28.5
Mobile	69.3	66.8	68.8	57.8

Sensory function, communication, and literacy – 6.5% of all residents in hospital had no useful vision; a further 10.3% were recorded as having very poor vision; 3.9% were deaf; a further 7.1% had poor hearing; 4.3% had a combination of visual and auditory handicaps; and 1.3% were both blind and deaf.

Of the residents in hospital, 40.5% could not speak at all, and a further 17.9% could only make their basic needs understood; 9.5% were rated as having no understanding at all, and 30.5% as having only basic understanding –

for example, they might have been able to understand the words or gestures for 'food' or 'sleep'.

The marked difference between the ability of some people with mental handicaps to understand and speak is apparent from the differences in these proportions. For many, the frustration of being unable to express even the most basic needs must be considerable, and may account for some of the behavioural problems.

Only a small proportion of the hospital residents were able to read (10.2%); 12.1% were able to make small purchases at the hospital or local shops; 6.9% were able to write brief letters or postcards when on holiday.

Self-help skills – overall, about 20% of the hospital residents were unable to feed themselves independently. About 40% could wash or dress themselves without help (Tables 6.9 and 6.10). The lack of ability to feed, wash, and dress is an indicator

Table 6.9 Hospital residents who are known to be unable to feed themselves or to need help with feeding according to age group (percentage)

Ability to feed self	Age group				
	15–29	30–44	45–64	> 64	Total
Not at all	14.4	11.1	6.8	2.9	8.8
With help	14.9	14.5	9.7	6.7	11.7
Feeds self	70.6	73.5	83.5	90.0	79.6
All	100.0	100.0	100.0	100.0	100.0

Table 6.10 Personal living skills of individuals living in hospital (%)

Skill	NK	Not at all	With help	Without help	All known
Feed self	20	129 (8.8)	172 (11.7)	1173 (79.6)	1474 (100)
Wash self	20	423 (28.6)	558 (37.8)	493 (33.4)	1474 (100)
Dress self	20	320 (21.7)	532 (36.1)	622 (42.2)	1474 (100)

of severe physical or intellectual handicap, or both. The proportion who were able to feed, wash, and dress themselves increased with increasing age. The most likely explanation, as with walking, is that those who were unable to feed, wash, and dress themselves were less likely to survive. The proportion of people with multiple disabilities in hospitals is high because many of the most able have already been resettled. Now only the most severely disabled are admitted. Thus, the nature of the hospital population is different from that of ten or more years ago.

Problems with behaviour

The classification, aggregation, and reasoning behind the collection of data about behaviour is outlined in Chapter 4. The same aggregation is followed in this chapter in order to make direct comparisons possible. The limitation of direct comparisons between the hospital group and residents elsewhere is that behaviours, which are tolerated on a large hospital ward, for example, noise, may not be acceptable within an inner-city flat. It is also likely that behavioural problems in hospital are appraised and reported differently in the hospital population, because of differences in expectations.

The percentage distribution of the hospital cases according to their rating for each of the behaviours is shown in Table 6.11.

Table 6.11 Behavioural problems according to severity – all individuals living in hospital (percentages)

Behaviour	Severe	Mild	None
Attention-seeking	9.2	22.9	67.9
Damaging property	9.0	21.6	74.0
Delinquent acts	4.5	12.5	83.1
Noise	14.7	28.1	57.1
Over-active	9.3	16.5	74.3
Objectionable habits	8.8	18.7	72.5
Personal aggression	13.6	25.9	60.5
Self-injury	7.9	15.7	76.4
Wandering off	5.8	14.6	79.6
Withdrawn	10.1	29.3	60.6

Table 6.12 Percentage with severe behavioural problems (often or occasional) by age group (residents in hospital only)

Behaviour	Age group				
	15–29	*30–44*	*45–64*	*65+*	*All*
Attention-seeking	17.9	11.3	6.0	3.7	9.2
Damaging property	20.2	11.8	4.4	2.9	9.0
Delinquent acts	7.2	5.3	3.1	2.8	4.5
Noise	24.2	16.6	11.6	8.8	14.7
Over-active	16.8	12.9	5.6	2.6	9.3
Objectionable habits	12.4	11.3	7.4	2.8	8.8
Personal aggression	27.8	17.8	7.8	4.5	13.6
Self-injury	15.7	10.7	5.3	0.7	7.9
Wandering off	10.8	6.8	4.3	2.4	5.8
Withdrawn	17.4	11.8	7.7	4.9	10.1

The most frequently recorded 'Severe' problems among hospital patients are noise (14.7%), personal aggression (13.6%), and being withdrawn (10.1%) (Table 6.12). Three other categories – over-activity, attention-seeking, and damaging property – each affect nearly 10%. The prevalence of all types of 'Severe' problems decreases with increasing age. In common with many of the problems that have been assessed, it is impossible to say whether this decrease in prevalence with age is the result of maturation or due to differential survival, differences in admission cohorts, or selective resettlement of the least severely affected individuals. An analysis of the archived data from the KCW register indicated that selective resettlement is the most likely (Farmer *et al.*, 1990).

Combinations of disabilities and problems

Of the hospital residents, 74.4% were recorded as having at least one 'Severe' behavioural or physical problem. Of the 1494 patients, (3.9%) 54 have more than three severe physical problems, and more than three severe behavioural problems (Table 6.13).

Table 6.13 Distribution of 'Severe physical' and 'Severe behavioural' problems among people living in hospitals aged >15 years, ( ) = percentages in each group

Number of severe physical problems	Number of severe behavioural problems				
	0	*1–2*	*3–5*	*>5*	Total
0	442 (29.6)	129 (8.6)	54 (3.6)	15 (1.0)	640
1–2	248 (16.6)	104 (7.0)	55 (3.7)	16 (1.1)	423
3–5	124 (8.3)	57 (3.8)	24 (1.6)	8 (0.5)	213
>5	152 (10.2)	39 (2.6)	19 (1.3)	8 (1.5)	218
Total	966	329	152	47	1494

Illustrative cases

Case E was a severely mentally handicapped 34-year-old woman, who had spina bifida and had lived in South Ockenden Hospital for 31 years. Her parents were still alive. She was doubly incontinent, could not wash herself at all, and needed help with dressing. She had no speech, and only basic understanding. She was fully mobile, but this constituted a problem because she had a tendency to wander. Her vision and hearing appeared to be normal. She was aggressive to people, damaged property, and was over-active. She had a tendency to injure herself, and was very noisy. Her personal habits were objectionable. She was recorded as requiring full-time support. During the day she had occupational therapy.

Case F was a young man who had lived in Bromham Hospital for 23 of his 24 years. He was profoundly mentally handicapped as a consequence of infection with *Escherichia coli*. He had epilepsy, which was only partially controlled with drugs, and he was doubly incontinent. Although he could walk with help, he used a wheelchair, with which he needed assistance. He needed help with feeding, and could not wash or dress himself at all. His vision and hearing appeared normal, but he had no speech and no apparent understanding. He had a tendency to damage property, and his personal habits were objectionable. He often became withdrawn and was sometimes noisy. His parents were still alive.

Case G was a 64-year-old man who was admitted to Fairfield Hospital when he was 50. He was deaf and mute, and blind. During the day he received occupational therapy. He could feed himself but could not dress himself. He could not communicate, but had some understanding. He was noisy and tended to damage property. Sometimes he was withdrawn. His next-of-kin was his brother.

Case H was a 27-year-old woman who had been in Leavesden Hospital for 18 years. She had the congenital rubella syndrome and was blind and deaf. She was doubly incontinent. She could feed herself and was fully mobile; could not wash herself but with help was able to dress. She tended to seek attention, injure herself, hit others, and damage property; sometimes she became withdrawn. During the day she attended a skills development unit in the hospital.

These cases are representative of the most disabled who were looked after in hospital. A very high percentage of all hospital patients had some major behavioural or physical problem that made them highly dependent upon others. It is likely that it will become increasingly difficult to find placements outside the hospital for many of those who remain.

Comparison of people living in hospitals with residents in all others places

People with mental handicaps resident in hospitals were more likely to have problems in all areas except vision, where the incidence of poor sight was less than that among people in other types of accommodation (Table 6.14). They did not

72

Table 6.14 Distribution of each of the variables for people living in hospital compared with all other people with mental handicaps (significant at $P < 0.01$)

Variable	Chi^2	Prob	Direction
Urinary incontinence/night	135.50	0.000	More
Faecal incontinence/night	169.35	0.000	More
Urinary incontinence/day	173.68	0.000	More
Faecal incontinence/day	142.77	0.000	More
Walking	267.43	0.000	More
Feeding	30.40	0.000	More
Washing	330.48	0.000	More
Dressing	213.11	0.000	More
Vision	74.04	0.000	Less
Hearing	10.43	0.005	More
Speech	388.13	0.000	More
Understanding	211.94	0.000	More
Personal aggression	109.85	0.000	More
Damaging	40.19	0.000	More
Over-active	8.92	NS	
Attention-seeking	3.12	NS	
Self-injury	36.58	0.000	More
Delinquent	52.63	0.000	More
Personal habits	177.22	0.000	More
Wandering	1.96	NS	
Noise	58.56	0.000	More

Less = Fewer severe problems among people living in hospital than all others on the registers.
More = More severe problems among people living in hospital than all others on the registers.

differ significantly from people in other residential categories in respect of damaging property, attention-seeking, and wandering off. The reasons they were not reported as having an excessive frequency of these behaviours may have been that the hospital environment in which they live is contrived to avoid these problems – for example, locks on wards that are difficult to operate, the use of indestructible furniture. Were they to have been located elsewhere, the picture might be different.

Summary

The hospitals for people with mental handicaps in the region are large, for example, Leavesden had 851 beds, Harperbury 730, Cell Barnes 520, and Bromham 298 beds. The residents were older than people who lived with their parents in the family home and those who lived in other types of residential provision. They had a higher incidence of physical and behavioural disorders. A very high percentage (70%) of the hospital residents had at least one behavioural problem.

The prevalence of physical disorders among the hospital residents was the highest of any of the residential groups. Severe difficulties in communication were reported in 54%, and severe problems with feeding in 21%.

The frequency of all problems was substantially higher in the hospital population than in any of the other residential categories. It appeared that the proportion affected had increased as the more able were transferred to community placements. This tendency has been further accentuated by death among the older hospital residents, some of whom were relatively able, and by the selective admission of only those with severe difficulties.

People with mental handicap who have physical and behavioural problems as well form one of the most difficult groups to care for. They are best described as multiply handicapped. They need higher staff-to-resident ratios, and greater technical skills among staff than any other group. Their environmental requirements need special consideration since many need aids and appliances, including appropriate wheelchairs and access for them. Many of the residents are intolerant of space restrictions. Virtually all in this group would be unsafe in open traffic.

As the proportion of multiply handicapped people in hospital rises, the staff ratio will have to increase to ensure an adequate standard of care. The resettlement of the most able from the hospital into the community will continue to increase the costs incurred in caring for the residual residents.

Summary

The process of closing the large mental handicap hospitals and relocating their patients in the community appeared to slow down or even to stop in some districts during the course of this investigation. Whatever policies eventually emerge, it is essential that people who are multiply handicapped have the benefit of trained specialists, working within properly organized systems, and that their particular medical, social, and environmental needs are met.

7

Residents in private or voluntary homes

Introduction

The private and voluntary (P/V) residential-care sector is of particular interest because current policy in the UK (HMSO: *Caring for People*, 1989) is based on an assumption that it should form the backbone of future provision. There is an important distinction between care provided privately and that provided by the voluntary, or charity, organizations.

The purely 'private' homes are established as businesses, with all the normal business constraints; they have to be managed profitably. There is nothing inherently wrong – or even undesirable – about providing care as a business, but it does have certain important consequences.

Inner urban properties are expensive to buy, to maintain and to staff. Unit costs are inevitably greater than those for equivalent properties in rural and suburban areas. Unless the paying authorities (normally the social services department of the LA of origin of the handicapped individual) recognize the differential costs by paying different rates for accommodation in different places, the tendency for private provision to be outside the main conurbations will continue. The present policy of many LAs is to seek the lowest cost, rather than the optimal geographical location of residence.

In the UK there is a long tradition of care for special groups of individuals being provided by the so-called 'voluntary sector'. Most of this is organized through registered national or local charities, many of which were formed by groups of committed individuals who recognized gaps in the services offered by the statutory authorities. The voluntary groups operate both as pressure groups and providers of innovative facilities for the people in whom they have a particular interest. Local MENCAP societies are particularly active in this field. Their survival and success is inevitably linked to the drive and long-term commitment of the individual members, and with their ability to raise funds to support their ventures.

The first task when planning residential facilities is to raise, or guarantee, the necessary capital. This is often achieved by a combination of charitable fund-raising activities – balls, fêtes, 'racing nights', bridge days, concerts, etc. – and personal guarantees of funds by members, charitable trusts, or wealthy benefactors. In the early stages of operation of a new residence, it is necessary to have sufficient independent funds to meet the running costs. Once the schemes are fully operational, the continued funding is usually made available by the statutory authorities on a similar basis to the funding of the private sector (a fixed amount per resident, per week).

Many of the voluntary organizations have specific objectives and target groups which reflect the concerns and enthusiasm of those who initiate the schemes. If the philosophy or type of provision required by the paying authorities moves too far from the original intent of the charities, then key individuals may become disillusioned. Disillusionment may endanger the survival of the organizations themselves. Clearly, it is essential that there should be close and sensitive relationships between the charities and the statutory authorities if the energy, enthusiasm, and commitment of parents and voluntary workers is to be fully realized. There will always be a potential for conflict between the underlying principles of the charity and the priorities set by the paying authority. The nature of the financial structure of the charities is such that the paying authority is often in a position to impose its own terms and philosophy.

As the P/V sectors are both substantially dependent on revenue funding from the statutory authorities, neither is in a position to risk expenditure in excess of their expected income. Thus, in general, some highly dependent people with mental handicaps are not accepted in this sector because the real costs of providing care is significantly in excess of the fees being offered. There is some indication that the situation is now changing as limited differential payments related to the level of disability are being negotiated in some areas. Clearly the size of the differentials will have to be substantial if these sectors are to provide for many of the severely disabled who are now in hospital, and those who would, in earlier times, have moved from their family home to a long-stay hospital.

Provision in NW Thames

Of the people with mental handicaps aged over 15 who originate from the area, 10.4% lived in accommodation provided privately or by the voluntary sector. The extent to which this type of provision was used varied greatly between districts. The area covered by the KCW register made the most extensive use of this sector (27.1%), and Hillingdon the least (0.5%) (Table 4.1).

Some of these differences may have been the result of differential registration according to the type of residence. However, it is unlikely to have been a major factor, since the estimated proportion of all people with mental handicaps who were registered was high for Hillingdon, and for some other authorities which had very small numbers of placements in the P/V sector. It is more likely that the observed differences reflected differences in policy between authorities – some were philosophically committed to providing all care within publicly owned and managed facilities, while others had more pragmatic approaches.

The geographical location of the accommodation in the P/V homes that were used by KCW outside the geographical boundaries of the authorities is shown in Figure 7.1. Many of the 'homes' were located considerable distances from the residents' districts of origin; some were even outside the region's boundaries. Their wide distribution posed two problems: it was difficult to monitor the quality of care provided, and it was difficult for the individuals to maintain contact with their families and communities. Many areas had no social-work time to cover either of these needs.

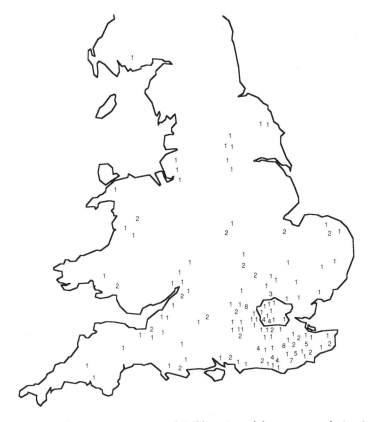

Figure 7.1 Approximate geographical location of the accommodation in P/V homes used by KCW and outside the borough of origin.

The residents

The residents in the P/V sector tended to be younger than those living in hospitals, and older than those living in their family homes. There was a significant expansion of the P/V sector in the mid-1980s. Their new residents came either from the hospitals or family homes. As the residents in this sector were relatively young, it is less likely that these places will be vacated by death than those in the hospitals. Once vacated by death, the hospital places will be closed permanently. It follows that there is a need to increase the provision in the P/V sector or in the LA sector, or both, to house those who can no longer live with their families.

Age and year of admission

Figure 7.2 shows the numbers of individuals who were living in this type of accommodation according to the year in which

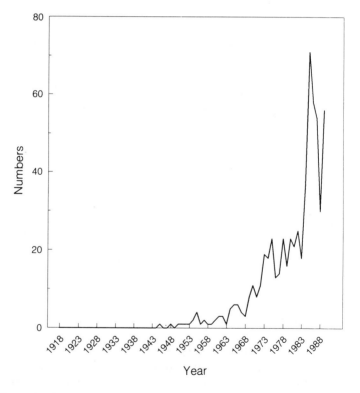

Figure 7.2 People with mental handicaps – residents in P/V accommodation by year of admission.

they were admitted. Clearly the numbers admitted many years previously had been reduced by death, thus the figures cannot be used to ascertain the actual numbers admitted in each of the years shown. The significant increase in numbers from the early 1980s onwards is unlikely to be explained by differences in mortality. The picture contrasts sharply with that for hospital admissions (Figure 6.2).

The majority who were living in the P/V sector had been admitted when they were in their late 'teens and early 20s (Figure 7.3). However, there was a change in the age distribution at admission of those admitted between 1975–84, and those admitted after 1985 (Table 7.1). The people more recently

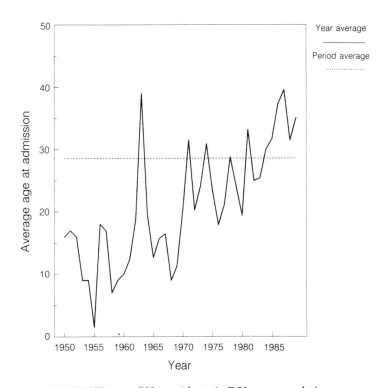

Figure 7.3 NW Thames RHA residents in P/V accommodation – average age at admission by year of admission.

Residents in private or voluntary homes

Table 7.1 Age distribution of people admitted to the P/V sector between 1975 and 1984 compared with those admitted in 1985 and later (percentages)

Admission period	Age at admission						
	0–19	20–29	30–39	40–49	50–59	60–	All
1975–84	47.7	21.8	11.1	10.6	6.9	1.9	100.0
1985–9	11.8	33.6	20.3	14.8	11.4	8.1	100.0

admitted were older. The most likely explanation for this is that the most recent cohort was recruited from the mental handicap hospital, whereas previous cohorts came directly from their own family homes or special boarding schools.

Day-time activity

About 90% of all residents in the P/V sector were involved in some formal activities during the day. The most frequently used occupation was attendance at an adult training centre, day centre, or social education centre. Among the 15–29-year-olds, a minority attended school. Less than 10% were employed either in sheltered workshops or elsewhere (Table 7.2). The small numbers in sheltered workshops may have been the result of there being insufficient places to meet the need, alternatively, it was possible that their disabilities precluded such activities.

Table 7.2 Day-time activities of people living in P/V homes and hostels (%)

Activity	15–29	30–44	45+	All
None	5.3	16.1	27.5	9.1
School	14.4	2.9	0.0	10.9
Attending college	3.7	2.2	0.0	3.1
Work experience	9.2	0.0	0.0	0.6
ATC, SEC, etc.	48.9	51.1	40.0	48.8
Sheltered employment	9.2	3.6	0.5	7.7
Open employment	0.9	0.7	0.0	0.8
Other	9.2	13.9	7.5	10.1
NK	7.6	9.5	20.0	8.8

Degree of mental handicap

The residents in P/V homes tended to be less severely handicapped than those living in hospital or in their family homes.
Overall, 39.9% of the P/V residents were said to be either
severely or profoundly mentally handicapped, compared with
62.2% of the hospital residents. This is likely to have been the
result of a combination of selection into this type of accommodation, and a selective discharge policy by the hospitals.

Abilities and disabilities

In marked contrast to the situation among hospital patients,
only a small proportion (less than 25%) of all residents had
any problems with incontinence (Table 7.3). The most
reasonable explanation for the difference is that people with
incontinence problems were not generally accepted in the P/V
sector.

Table 7.3 Assessment of continence – residents in P/V homes and hostels
> 15 years of age, ( )= percentages of those known

Continence	NK	Frequent	Occasional	Never
Urinary/day	11	35 (5.8)	92 (15.3)	475 (78.9)
Urinary/night	11	41 (7.4)	100 (16.6)	461 (76.6)
Faecal/day	15	22 (3.7)	63 (10.5)	513 (85.8)
Faecal/night	16	22 (3.7)	50 (8.4)	525 (87.9)

Table 7.4 Residents in P/V homes with mobility problems according to
age group (percentages)

Ability to walk	Age group				
	15–29	30–44	45–64	> 64	Total
NK	1.7	1.0	0.7	0.0	1.1
Not at all	8.4	3.5	5.1	0.0	5.5
With help	4.2	4.5	4.4	15.0	5.1
Mobile	69.3	66.8	68.8	57.8	88.3
All	100.0	100.0	100.0	100.0	100.0

Of residents, 88.3% were fully mobile (Table 7.4), compared with 67.1% of those residents in hospital, and 76.3% living in their family homes. In general, the admission policy to P/V homes tended to exclude those with mobility problems, either because they did not have sufficient level access, or because they could not provide the level of staffing necessary.

Sensory function, communication, and literacy

Of the residents in P/V homes, 2.0% had no useful vision; a further 16.0% had poor vision; 3.4% were deaf; 7.0% of the residents had poor hearing; 3.8% had a combination of visual and hearing handicaps; 0.7% were both deaf and blind.

For 16.2%, their only use of speech was to communicate their basic needs and 14.8% could not speak at all. This compares dramatically with the residents in hospital, 40.5% of whom were unable to speak. This difference in the degree of disability of the group resident in P/V homes and of those resident in hospitals is demonstrated again in the small percentage who were recorded as having no understanding (2.4%) – compared to 9.5% in the hospitals – and of those who only had basic understanding (19.5%) – compared to 30.5% in the hospitals.

The greater overall ability of residents in the P/V homes compared with hospital patients was reflected in the proportion able to read (19.0%), to write a brief letter or postcard (14.2%), and to make small purchases (17.8%).

Self-help skills

The self-help skills of those living in P/V homes (Table 7.5) were greater than those of the hospital patients (Table 6.9). Although the people living in P/V accommodation were generally more able than the hospital population, there was a proportion who had considerable needs for support. One-third either needed help with washing themselves or could not wash themselves at all; one-quarter needed help with dressing or could not dress themselves at all.

Table 7.5 Personal living skills of individuals living in P/V homes

Skill	NK	Not at all	With help	Without help	All
Feed self	8 (1.1%)	14 (2.3%)	44 (7.2%)	547 (89.2%)	613 (100%)
Wash self	9 (1.5%)	41 (6.7%)	149 (24.3%)	414 (67.5%)	613 (100%)
Dress self	9 (1.5%)	38 (6.2%)	125 (20.4%)	441 (71.9%)	613 (100%)

Behavioural problems

The most frequently recorded 'Severe' problems in behaviour among those in P/V homes were being withdrawn (8.1%), noisy (7.9%), and seeking attention (7.7%) (Table 7.6). Three other categories – damage to property, over-activity, and aggression to persons – each affected just over 5%. Few of the severely behaviourally disturbed were accommodated in the P/V sector.

Table 7.6 Behavioural problems according to severity of all those living in P/V accommodation (percentages)

Behaviour	Severe	Mild	None
Attention-seeking	7.7	24.7	67.8
Damaging property	5.5	15.6	78.8
Delinquent acts	3.3	13.2	83.5
Noise	7.9	27.8	64.3
Over-active	5.9	19.5	74.5
Objectionable personal habits	3.8	13.1	83.1
Personal aggression	6.6	25.5	67.9
Self-injury	3.9	12.8	83.2
Wandering off	3.6	15.3	81.1
Withdrawn	8.1	37.0	54.8

Combinations of disabilities and problems

There were very few people who had more than three problems on both axes (Table 7.7). The vast majority had either no severe problems or one to two on either axis (80.5%).

Table 7.7 Distribution of 'Severe physical' and 'Severe behavioural' problems among people aged > 15 years living in P/V homes and hostels, ( ) = percentages in each group

No. of severe physical problems	No. of severe behavioural problems				
	0	1–2	3–5	>5	Total
0	347 (56.6)	53 (8.6)	20 (3.3)	7 (1.1)	429
1–2	94 (15.3)	28 (4.6)	8 (1.3)	4 (0.6)	134
3–5	18 (2.9)	6 (1.0)	5 (0.8)	0 (0.0)	29
>5	17 (2.8)	3 (0.5)	0 (0.0)	1 (0.2)	21
Total	476	92	33	12	613

Illustrative case

In previous chapters, a selection of the most severely affected individuals have been described in some detail. There was only one individual in the P/V sector who complied with the selection criteria used in the chapter on hospital residents and on residents in family homes.

Case I was a young man of 18 years, who had lived in a children's home since he was nine. His next-of-kin was his mother; there was no mention of his father. Profoundly mentally handicapped, he was also doubly incontinent, needed help with feeding, and was unable to either wash or dress himself. Both his vision and hearing were poor. He had no speech and only basic understanding. He was fully independently mobile, but this caused a problem as he was prone to wander off. He was aggressive, over-active, had objectionable personal habits, and was noisy. Clearly, the time he would be able to continue to live in an institution for children was limited. The pattern of his problems was more like that associated with hospital patients than with adults in the private or voluntary sector.

Table 7.8 Distribution of each of the variables for people living in P/V homes and hostels compared with all others with mental handicaps (significant at P < 0.01)

Variable	Chi^2	Prob	Direction
Urinary incontinence/night	32.57	0.000	Less
Faecal incontinence/night	25.49	0.000	Less
Urinary incontinence/day	15.71	0.000	Less
Faecal incontinence/day	17.44	0.000	Less
Walking	28.98	0.000	Less
Feeding	20.60	0.000	Less
Washing	70.59	0.000	Less
Dressing	62.91	0.000	Less
Vision	4.21	NS	
Hearing	1.77	NS	
Speech	18.19	0.000	Less
Understanding	6.68	NS	
Personal aggression	14.53	0.006	Less
Damaging	5.11	NS	
Over-active	4.05	NS	
Attention-seeking	38.77	0.000	More
Self-injury	6.97	NS	
Delinquent	16.83	0.002	More
Objectional personal habits	3.08	NS	
Wandering	7.63	NS	
Noise	8.69	NS	
Withdrawn	22.88	0.000	More

Less = Fewer severe problems among people living in P/V homes than all others on the registers.
More = More severe problems among people living in P/V homes than all others on the registers.

Comparison of people living in P/V accommodation with residents in other places

Residents in P/V establishments were generally less disabled and had fewer behavioural problems than those who lived elsewhere (Table 7.8). Specifically, they had fewer problems with incontinence, walking, feeding, washing, dressing, speech, and personal aggression. As a group they tended to seek attention and exhibit delinquent behaviour more than people in other residences. This may have been because the environment offered opportunities that were not available elsewhere. On the other hand, both of these parameters are judgemental, and the relatively high scores might reflect the expectations of those who made the assessments. A significantly higher proportion of the residents of P/V establishments were withdrawn.

The overall picture is consistent with a high degree of selectivity into P/V accommodation. A relatively homogeneous group is identifiable. The traditional role of this type of establishment has been to care for the most able; it appears this tradition has been maintained.

Summary

The data clearly illustrates that the people who were living in P/V accommodation had greater abilities in daily-living skills than those who were living in family homes or in hospitals. The relative lack of aggressive and destructive behaviour among the group living in P/V accommodation was marked – this has important implications, since these are the behaviours which require the greatest levels of staff skill and time.

The 1989 White Paper *Caring for People* envisaged the P/V sector as the principal provider of residential places for the majority of people with mental handicaps. The fact that this sector now provides care for the least disabled gives cause for concern. A large number of the people who currently live in other types of accommodation, for example, those in hospitals or in their family homes, would not be suitable for the type of places now offered by the P/V sector. These places are staffed on the assumption that the residents will be able to care for themselves to a certain extent, and will not have major behavioural problems or significant physical needs.

A change in the nature of the accommodation provided in this sector has cost implications. Unless they are recognized and financed, the government's plans may not be achieved. The costs of caring for people with combinations of challenging behaviours, psychiatric, and medical problems escalates dramatically as the number and severity of the problems in a particular individual increases.

The problems of monitoring quality will become more difficult when people with complex needs are involved. It is further complicated by a significant proportion of the P/V homes being sited in areas which are not easily accessible to those who are responsible for and paying for the residents. Moreover, the success of much of the accommodation in the P/V sector is dependent on LA day care, which is outside the control of either the paying authority or the providers of the accommodation. These issues came to light in the course of several enquiries, see for example, St Bernard's (1990) and Bromley (1989).

It is clear that the policies of 'community care' need further detailed consideration and costing before people with complex and multiple handicaps can be offered placements in P/V facilities.

8

Residents in Local Authority homes and hostels

Introduction

In England and Wales, the local government authorities (LAs), through their social service departments, provide accommodation and care for certain groups with special needs – these include the elderly, people with physical handicaps, chronic mental illness, and some people with mental handicaps. The level of provision varies considerably between authorities, and depends on local traditions, local priorities, and the availability of resources. Most LA group homes and hostels are located within the geographical boundaries of the authority.

Government policy as set out in *Care in the Community* (1989) envisaged the care of people with mental handicaps being funded through either the LAs or the health service, but that ideally it should not be provided by either. The policy placed the LAs who had made some provision in a slightly difficult position. They continue to provide accommodation and other facilities, but it is unlikely they will be prepared to invest much more capital for residential care until the statutory situation is clarified. In the meantime, the policy of authorities varies.

Provision in NW Thames

Between 5–18% of people with mental handicaps in the NW Thames region lived in LA hostel and group home accommo-

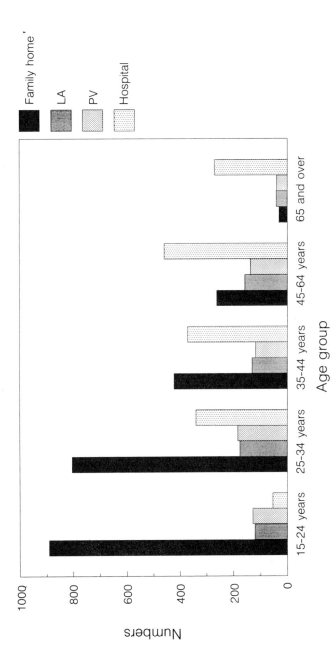

Figure 8.1 People with mental handicaps – numbers in each age group in LA compared with other accommodation.

dation, depending on which LA was responsible for them. In common with those people who lived in P/V accommodation, they tended to be younger than people with mental handicaps who lived in hospital, and older than those who lived in their family homes (Figure 8.1).

The distribution of residents in LA accommodation according to length of stay was similar to that of residents in P/V homes and hostels (Figure 8.2). This reflects the change in policy in the late 1960s, whereby there was a general shift of emphasis from hospital to community care with a consequent increase in the volume of non-hospital accommodation. Surprisingly, no real change in the average age at admission to LA establishments is apparent over the last 25 years

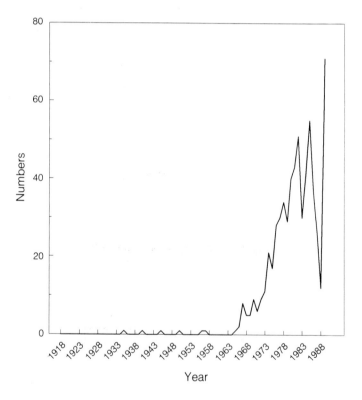

Figure 8.2 People with mental handicaps – residents in LA accommodation by year of admission.

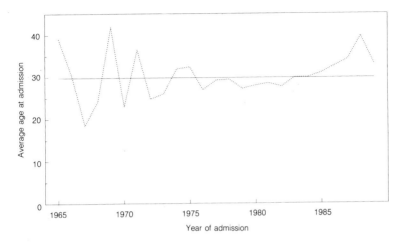

Figure 8.3 People with mental handicaps – residents in LA accommodation – average age at admission by year of admission.

(Figure 8.3). In earlier years, most of the admissions were from family homes, but more recently they have been from hospitals.

Degree of mental handicap

Of those living in LA homes, whose degree of mental handicap was known, 30.9% were recorded as being severely or profoundly mentally handicapped. This is a smaller proportion than those who were living in hospital (62.2%). The distribution of the residents of LA homes and hostels according to the degree of mental handicap is virtually the same as those who live in P/V accommodation. Like the P/V homes, the LAs tended to avoid taking the most severely handicapped because their staffing levels were not appropriate. The most dependent people were seen as the responsibility of the health service.

Day-time activity

The day-time activity of those who were resident in LA-owned and managed residential accommodation is shown in Table 8.1. A higher proportion were involved in some day-time activity than was the case for residents in the P/V sector.

Table 8.1 Day-time activities of people living in LA homes and hostels

	Age group			
Activity	*15–29*	*30–44*	*45+*	*All*
None	1.7	0.0	12.6	4.6
School	23.0	0.0	0.0	8.2
Home teaching	0.0	0.5	1.5	0.6
Attending college	3.5	3.9	0.0	2.5
Work experience	0.0	0.5	0.5	0.3
ATC, SEC, etc.	57.1	83.5	72.4	70.5
Sheltered employment	0.4	0.5	0.0	0.3
Open employment	1.3	3.4	2.5	2.4
Other	2.2	1.0	4.5	2.5
NK	10.6	6.8	6.0	7.9

The ATCs, SECs, and similar centres provided the bulk of day care. Only 4.6% had no day activity. This contrasts markedly with the hospital population, where over 30% had none. This was the result of the relatively greater use of SECs and ATCs by the LAs for their own residents.

Abilities and disabilities

Table 8.2 shows that, as with those who were living in P/V accommodation, most of the residents were continent (76.1%);

Table 8.2 Assessment of continence – residents in LA homes and hostels > 15 years of age, ( ) = percentages of those known

	NK	*Frequent*	*Occasional*	*Never*
Urinary/day	62	32 (5.6)	75 (13.1)	462 (81.2)
Urinary/night	61	58 (10.2)	78 (13.7)	434 (76.1)
Faecal/day	63	25 (4.4)	52 (9.1)	491 (86.4)
Faecal/night	65	21 (3.7)	51 (9.0)	494 (87.2)

Table 8.3 Residents in LA homes with mobility problems according to age group (percentages)

Ability to walk	Age group				
	15–29	*30–44*	*45–64*	*>64*	Total
NK	10.2	7.8	5.1	9.8	8.1
Not at all	10.6	4.4	3.2	4.9	5.5
With help	3.5	4.8	4.4	4.9	5.1
Mobile	75.7	83.0	87.3	61.0	81.3

81.3% were fully mobile (Table 8.3). This is very similar to the proportion in P/V homes (88.3%), and represented a higher proportion than those who lived in hospital (67.1%). The difference was probably due to a selective admission policy, necessitated by their staffing levels and the lack of level access.

Sensory function, communication, and literacy

Of the residents in LA homes, 2.5% had no useful vision, and a further 13.1% had poor vision; 1.7% were deaf; and 6.6% were regarded as having poor hearing. Only one person was both blind and deaf, but some 3.6% had a combination of visual and hearing handicaps; 14.2% could not speak at all, and a further 12.0% could only communicate at a basic level. This proportion, although very similar to that for people who were resident in P/V homes, is quite different to that of the hospital population, 40.5% of whom could not speak at all.

Of residents, 16.3% are able to read, 11.9% to write brief notes or letters, and 16.5% to count, to the extent that they can make small purchases. They are a more able group than those in hospital, and similar to those living in P/V accommodation.

Self-help skills

The level of self-help skills of those living in LA accommodation

Table 8.4 Personal living skills of individuals living in LA homes

Skill	NK	Not at all	With help	Without help	All
Feed self	57 (9.0)	16 (2.5)	43 (6.8)	515 (81.6)	631 (100)
Wash self	58 (9.2)	44 (6.9)	122 (19.3)	407 (64.5)	631 (100)
Dress self	58 (9.2)	41 (6.4)	103 (16.3)	429 (68.0)	631 (100)

(Table 8.4) was similar to that for residents in P/V homes, and greater than that of those in hospital (Table 6.10). Although only 2.5% could not feed themselves at all, and 6.8% needed help with feeding, about one-third needed help with washing and dressing.

Behavioural problems

The most frequently recorded 'Severe' behavioural problem was aggression towards people. Attention-seeking, damaging property, noise, over-activity, and being withdrawn each affects between 5–10% (Table 8.5). People who were living in

Table 8.5 Behavioural problems according to severity of all those living in LA accommodation (percentages)

Behaviour	Severe	Mild	None
Attention-seeking	8.2	30.0	61.7
Damaging property	7.4	12.5	80.0
Delinquent acts	4.8	13.9	81.3
Noise	9.6	28.5	61.9
Over-active	6.3	16.5	77.2
Objectionable personal habits	3.9	14.9	81.2
Personal aggression	10.9	23.8	65.3
Self-injury	4.8	12.7	82.5
Wandering off	2.8	12.2	84.9
Withdrawn	8.6	34.7	56.7

LA accommodation were slightly more likely to have had severe behavioural problems than were those living in P/V homes (Table 7.6).

Combinations of disabilities and problems

As seen in Table 8.6, 43.2% had one or more severe physical or behavioural problems. This is similar to the proportion found in P/V homes (43.4%), and very different from the proportion found in hospital (70.4%). The distribution of residents according to the severity of their physical and behavioural problems is shown in Table 8.6. No individual had a score of more than five on both axes, and only 1.0% had three or more problems on both axes. Most had no severe problems.

Table 8.6 Distribution of 'Severe physical' and 'Severe behavioural' problems among people aged > 15 years living in LA homes and hostels, ( ) = percentages in each group

No. severe physical problems	No. severe behavioural problems				
	0	1–2	3–5	>5	Total
0	365 (57.8)	57 (9.0)	20 (3.2)	6 (1.0)	448
1–2	80 (12.6)	36 (5.7)	10 (1.5)	4 (0.6)	130
3–5	17 (2.6)	6 (1.0)	6 (1.0)	1 (0.2)	30
>5	18 (2.9)	4 (0.6)	2 (0.2)	0 (0.0)	23
Total	480	103	37	11	631

Illustrative case

There was only one individual within the LA sector who had both severe physical and behavioural problems. This person was not as physically disabled as the people used as illustrative cases in the chapters on family home or hospital residents.

Case J was a 20-year-old man affected with epilepsy. He was rated as severely mentally handicapped. Doubly incontinent, he needed help with dressing, could not speak, but had good understanding. He was rated as having severe problems in all the measures of behaviour.

Comparison of people living in LA accommodation with residents in other places

People with mental handicaps who lived in LA accommodation were generally less physically disabled and had fewer behavioural problems than those residing elsewhere (Table 8.7).

Table 8.7 Distribution of each of the variables for people living in LA homes and hostels compared with all others with mental handicaps (significant at $P < 0.01$)

Variable	Chi^2	Prob	Direction
Urinary incontinence/night	6.62	NS	
Faecal incontinence/night	11.89	0.003	Less
Urinary incontinence/day	9.88	0.007	Less
Faecal incontinence/day	8.55	NS	
Walking	15.96	0.000	Less
Feeding	8.95	NS	
Washing	56.80	0.000	Less
Dressing	39.93	0.000	Less
Vision	1.08	NS	
Hearing	0.15	NS	
Speech	4.70	NS	
Understanding	9.30	0.010	Less
Personal aggression	10.11	NS	
Damaging	6.14	NS	
Over-active	1.13	NS	
Attention-seeking	13.17	0.010	More
Self-injury	3.35	NS	
Delinquent	22.81	0.000	More
Objectionable personal habits	11.57	NS	
Wandering	2.03	NS	
Noise	6.22	NS	

Less = Fewer severe problems among people living in LA homes and hostels than all others on the registers.
More = More severe problems among people living in LA homes and hostels than all others on the registers.

They were, however, more likely to exhibit attention-seeking and 'delinquent' behaviours. Both of these indices involve some degree of value judgement, and their relatively high scores may reflect the expectations of those responsible for providing care, rather than real differences between groups.

It is noteworthy that this group had a significantly lower prevalence of incontinence, difficulties in walking, dressing, and understanding. The most likely explanation for this is selection of entry to the establishments.

Summary

The characteristics of the residents in LA accommodation were remarkably similar to those of the people who lived in P/V accommodation. They were more able than those who lived in hospital or in their family homes. This was the result of specific selection policies. In the past, LA accommodation was designed for the most able; those with high levels of disability were the responsibility of the health service.

Most residents in LA accommodation were continent (76%); able to walk (81%); to speak well (74%); and had self-help skills (64%). There were 57.8% with no severe physical or behavioural problems – a similar proportion to those in P/V accommodation (56.6%).

Current policy encourages LAs to contract the provision of residential care to P/V agencies rather than to provide the services themselves. The scheme seems workable – the group currently cared for in the P/V sector closely matches the group living in LA accommodation. However, a problem is now becoming apparent: both the P/V and LA sectors are expected to accommodate a more disabled group – including people being 'resettled' from hospital and those who previously would have been admitted to hospital. The considerable uncertainties about funding make it unlikely that there will be any enthusiasm on the part of the P/V agencies to provide care for the severely disabled. This may result in the LAs both having to expand their level of provision and change their character. Alternatively, the current hospital closure programme will have to be curtailed.

9

Residents in NHS hostels

Introduction

The NHS provides two broad types of hostel accommodation, one sort is usually on, or close to, the mental handicap hospital campus. Such hostels are used for more able 'patients' in order to give them a more congenial way of life within the context of a secure setting. Recently some have been used as 'half-way houses' to train people for eventual resettlement in the community. In many hostels of this type, staff are shared with the main hospital. More recently, a new sort of specialist unit has been developed by health authorities. These units provide care for people with multiple and severe handicaps, and are separate from the hospitals. The residents receive hospital-type care in modern purpose-built accommodation. They are smaller in scale and more home-like than the hospitals. Some such hostels are located in the grounds of non-mental-handicap hospitals, within the geographical area they serve.

Provision in NW Thames

Eighty-two people, 1.4% of those registered, lived in this type of accommodation. Roughly half were in high-dependency units, and the other half were in relatively low-dependency accommodation. Over half were under 30 years of age.

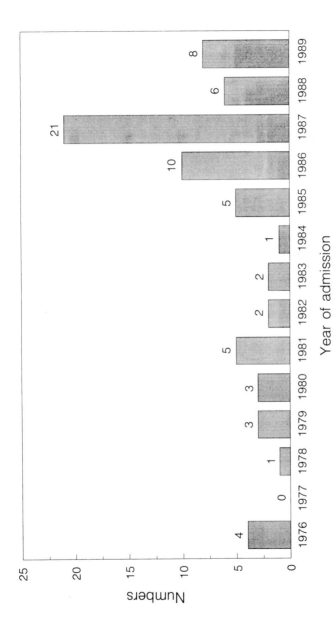

Figure 9.1 Residents in NHS hostels year of admission since 1976.

The majority of the residents in NHS hostels came from three geographical areas: KCW 28 (34%); Hammersmith and Fulham 23 (28%); and Brent 15 (18%). Each of these areas had NHS hostels within their geographical boundaries. The small numbers from the other registers might have been because they remain registered at the hospitals within which the hostels are located, rather than being separately recorded. Most of the people in this group had been transferred to hostel accommodation since the early 1980s (Figure 9.1). In the mid-1980s there was a sharp rise in the average age at admission (Figure 9.2), this was probably the result of a change in policy.

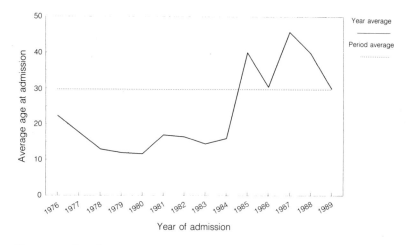

Figure 9.2 Residents in NHS hostels – average age at admission by year of admission.

Degree of handicap

Less than 10% of the residents in NHS hostels were rated as profoundly handicapped – 21.7% of the hospital residents were profoundly handicapped. The 'Mild' and 'Moderate' categories represented 39%.

Abilities and disabilities

Of all residents in NHS hostels, 51.2% had some sort of problem with incontinence; 18.2% could not walk at all; and a further 8.5% needed help with walking; 6.1% were blind, and 6.1% were deaf; 12.2% had some visual and auditory handicaps. Two were completely blind and deaf; 42.7% could not speak at all, and a further 18.3% could only make their basic needs known.

Mobility and self-help

The high disabilty levels of some of the groups living in NHS hostels is demonstrated in the proportion who could not feed themselves at all (13.4%), and a further 13.4% who needed help with feeding; 53.7% either could not wash themselves at all or needed help to wash; and 56.1% needed to be dressed or needed help dressing.

Behavioural problems

The levels and frequency of behavioural problems among the NHS hostel residents was similar to that of the hospital residents (Table 9.1).

Table 9.1 Behavioural problems, according to severity, of all individuals living in NHS hostels (percentages)

Behaviour	Severe	Mild	None
Attention-seeking	15.1	22.8	62.0
Damaging property	11.3	20.0	68.8
Delinquent acts	3.4	7.6	88.6
Noise	12.5	20.0	65.7
Over-active	6.3	15.2	78.5
Objectionable personal habits	5.1	12.7	82.3
Personal aggression	11.3	23.8	65.0
Self-injury	8.8	15.0	76.3
Wandering off	6.3	11.3	82.5
Withdrawn	10.1	22.8	67.1

Epilepsy

Thirteen of the 82 NHS hostel residents were affected with epilepsy. In all but one case it was either controlled or partially controlled.

Combinations of disabilities and problems

Table 9.2 shows the combinations of severe problems experienced by residents in NHS hostels. A greater proportion (32.9%) than those living in hospital had no severe problems, but the distinct characteristics of the two groups served by NHS hostels is demonstrated by the larger proportion who had five or more severe physical problems (15.8%).

Table 9.2 Distribution of 'severe physical' and 'severe behavioural' problems amongst people living in NHS hostels aged > 15 years, ( ) = percentages in each group

Number of severe physical problems	Number of severe behavioural problems				
	0	1–2	3–5	>5	Total
0	27 (32.9)	9 (11.0)	2 (2.4)	1 (1.2)	39
1–2	10 (12.2)	6 (7.3)	2 (2.4)	1 (1.2)	19
3–5	3 (3.6)	2 (2.4)	3 (3.6)	0	8
>5	13 (15.8)	1 (1.2)	1 (1.2)	1 (1.2)	16
Total	53	18	8	3	82

Illustrative cases

The marked difference in the type of person found in NHS hostels can be illustrated by two contrasting cases. The first is a relatively able person who was destined to be resettled in the community. He was using the NHS hostel as a half-way house. The second is a person who had been placed in a specialist NHS hostel because the multiplicity and difficulty of her problems meant she would not have been able to be admitted either to LA or to P/V accommodation.

Case K was a 58-year-old man who lived in one of the NHS hostels attached to and run by St Lawrence's Hospital. He originated from Westminster, but had no next-of-kin. He was described as mildly mentally handicapped. There were no causal or complicating diagnoses recorded. He was continent, and fully able in self-help skills. He could speak well, and, although he could not read at all, he could understand money and sign his name. He was in sheltered employment. He could use the telephone, travel on public transport, and socialize independently. He needed some help with shopping. There were no behavioural problems described.

Case L lived in a specialist unit and originated from Brent. She was a young woman of 17 whose parents were alive. She had lived in the unit for eight years. She was described as profoundly mentally handicapped. The cause of her mental handicap was meningitis, and she was quadriplegic. She also had epilepsy and asthma. Doubly incontinent, she could not walk or manage her wheelchair. She could not feed, wash, or dress herself at all, and her vision and hearing were described as poor. She had no speech, and no observable evidence of understanding. There were no behavioural problems recorded. She attended a special day-care unit.

Summary

Residents in NHS hostels fell into two distinct groups: a group of relatively able people who had spent much of ther lives in hospital and who were now using the NHS hostels as a stepping-stone to the community; and a group of multiply handicapped individuals who were difficult to place in P/V or LA accommodation because of their level of disability. The first group is comparable to residents in P/V accommodation; the second is comparable to the most disabled in family homes or in hospitals.

In planning terms, the second group is of particular interest as they may be the only group for whom the NHS will provide residential accommodation in the future. Their needs are high, and a high level of staff skill and commitment is required. Many of these residents had serious difficulties in feeding and mobility – both of which are associated with premature death (Eyman, 1990).

Policies and funding arrangements for the provision of residential and day care for people with multiple and severe handicaps have not yet been formulated. About 25% of people with mental handicaps come into this category – they are cared for mainly at home or in hospital. A few live in NHS hostels or special P/V units. This most vulnerable group, for whom the cost of care is high, still await an achievable plan for the 1990s.

10

Residents in other types of institution

There remains a group of people who live in a variety of types of accommodation other than those described earlier in this book. Each type is, in its own way, a fascinating example of the variety of provision which has evolved in an attempt to encompass the needs of people with mental handicaps. They include 'foster homes', group homes, religious establishments, old people's homes, and sheltered housing. A few live independently.

The ages of the people who lived in the type of accommodation covered in this chapter are shown in Figure 10.1. They are, on the whole, younger than those who resided in hospitals, LA or P/V residential accommodation, but were older than those who lived in their family homes.

Some attempts have been made to settle selected individuals in foster homes within the community. A 'foster' home is a normal household in which one or more of the members agree to accept an individual as a 'member of the family', for payment by one or other of the statutory authorities. The arrangement is regarded as permanent while the key household member is able to cope. Sixty-one adults with mental handicaps in NW Thames were being 'fostered'. They were mostly young (over half of them being under 30 years); 19 of them attended day schools; and the majority of the remainder attended SECs. Two people were in open employment. Six had no day-time activity (Table 10.1). There were no profoundly mentally handicapped people in foster homes. Most of the fostered individuals

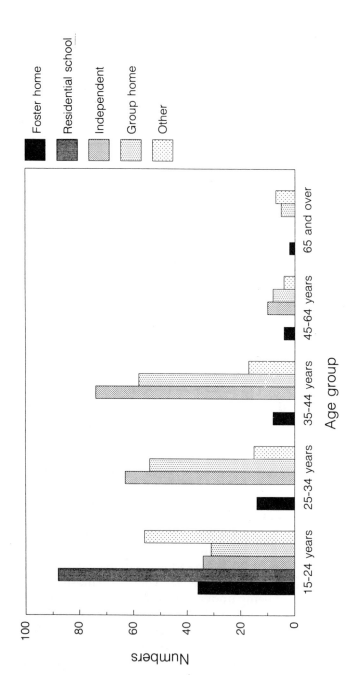

Figure 10.1 People with mental handicaps – numbers in each age group in different types of residential accommodation.

Table 10.1 Principal day activities of those in all other types of residence

	Foster home	Resid. school	Indep.	Group home	Other	Total
None	6	1	44	21	5	77
Day school	19	2	0	1	32	54
Boarding school	2	62	0	0	0	64
Home teaching	0	0	0	0	1	1
College	0	8	7	9	3	27
Work experience	0	0	4	2	0	6
ATC/SEC	24	0	60	70	17	171
Sheltered employ	0	1	5	10	1	17
Open employment	2	0	29	20	0	51
Other	1	0	17	5	0	23
NK	7	11	15	18	37	88
All	61	85	181	156	96	579

Table 10.2 Degree of mental handicap of people living in all other accommodation

	Foster home	Resid. school	Indep.	Group home	Other	Total
Using MH servs	6	7	37	27	4	81
ICD code						
317 Mild m. ret.	7	11	91	62	13	184
318.0 Mod. m. ret.	13	13	19	30	5	80
318.1 Sev. m. ret.	13	16	1	7	16	53
318.2 Prof. m. ret.	0	1	0	0	1	2
319 Unspec. m. ret.	19	33	29	27	34	142
NK	1	3	3	1	23	31
Total	61	85	181	156	96	579

had a mild or moderate handicap; six were described simply as 'using mental handicap services'. (Table 10.2).

Most in foster homes were fully continent, only four had frequent urinary incontinence, and two frequent faecal incontinence. A further 13 had occasional problems with incontinence. The proportion of people who are incontinent was similar to that found in family homes; 87.7% of people in foster homes could walk unaided; three people could not manage stairs; and four are unable to walk at all.

One fostered person had no useful vision, and nine had poor vision. One was deaf and three others had hearing problems. Most people in foster homes could speak well, although there were six who had no speech and five who could only communicate their basic needs. All were described as having some level of observable understanding; in six people this was described as 'Basic'. Literacy skills are shown in Table 10.3.

Most people in foster homes were able to feed themselves (Table 10.4). Many needed help with washing (nearly one-third), and seven people were unable to wash themselves. A similar proportion needed help with dressing.

Table 10.3 Percentage with some literacy skills – individuals living in all other residences

	Type of residence				
Skill	*Foster home*	*Resid. school*	*Indep.*	*Group home*	*Other*
Read or write a little	53.7	59.5	88.0	77.4	55.8
Write or sign name	59.3	65.3	90.4	77.4	53.5
Understand money or count	73.5	75.6	95.8	92.5	65.1

Table 10.4 Percentage with self-help skills – individuals living in all other residences

	Type of residence				
Able to	*Foster home*	*Resid. school*	*Indep.*	*Group home*	*Other*
Feed self	83.6	89.3	99.4	99.3	84.1
Wash self	58.2	58.1	96.0	97.9	60.4
Dress self	63.6	55.4	98.3	97.3	58.1

Of those living with foster parents, 87.5% had no severe behavioural problems. The most frequently recorded problem was 'attention-seeking', one person had five severe behavioural problems recorded. It seems as though on the whole, more able individuals were being fostered, however, among them were some multiply handicapped individuals.

Another option for residential care for young people is the residential school. There were 85 young people over the age of 15 years who were at residential schools. Although most received their education at the school, there were eight individuals who attended 'college', one was in 'sheltered employment', and two were attending day school, presumably away from the residential facility.

The day-time activity of 11 was not known. These were somewhat surprising findings. It might be expected that all pupils at a residential school would be attending classes during the day. Some of these young people remain in the residential schools after formal classroom education has been completed in order to extend their experience while remaining in a familiar environment. For some there is nowhere else to go.

Only one of the residential school pupils was profoundly mentally handicapped. A large proportion (40%) were described as having an 'unspecified mental retardation' (ICD 319) (Table 10.2), thus the proportions in the categories 'Mild', 'Moderate', 'Severe', and 'Profound' may not be a true reflection of the whole group.

Most of the young people in residential schools were continent (74.0%), however, 19 (26%) had frequent or occasional incontinence at night; 93.2% could walk unaided; one person had no useful vision, and a further 11 (14.7%) had poor vision, even when wearing spectacles. One person was deaf, and a further eight (10.7%) had problems with hearing; 64.9% had good speech, but 15 (20.3%) could not speak at all. All were described as having some level of understanding.

The proportion of pupils at residential schools who had some degree of literacy is shown in Table 10.3. It is not as high as for those who lived independently or those in group homes, but over half (59.5%) could read a little, and a larger proportion could write or count. These are skills that are essential to survival in the community – in normal life people need to be able to read signs or understand pictograms, make small purchases, and sign their name for a variety of minor transactions. Residential schools seem to have taught these skills successfully to a large proportion of the pupils selected for entry.

Most (89.3%) could feed themselves, but 40% needed help with washing themselves, and 42% needed help with dressing (Table 10.4). The majority (58%) of the pupils had no severe behavioural problems; 25% had more than two severe problems, and one individual had nine severe problems. Of the behavioural problems, noise, attention-seeking, over-activity, and withdrawn behaviour were problems in more than 20% of pupils in residential schools, while personal aggression, self-injury and damaging property was a problem in 15–20%.

It is clear that the residential schools were taking young people with a high level of behavioural disturbance. The proportion of severe physical problems was not great – 71.8% had no severe problem and only five (5.9%) had more than two severe problems. In earlier times, some of these children might have been admitted to hospital care because their behavioural problems were such that their families would not have been able to contain them.

The numbers of young people with severe, or moderately severe, behavioural problems in residential schools represents a potential problem. There were and still are not, sufficient numbers of specialized residential establishments outside the hospitals that are equipped and staffed to accept adults with the levels of behavioural disturbance found in this group.

One-hundred-and-eighty-one people lived independent lives. The term 'independent' when used in this context needs some explanation. Most individuals with mental handicaps who lived 'independently' were receiving a considerable amount of help and support from social workers – often these were the social workers attached to the residential service from which 'independent' individuals had been rehoused. They were also supported by 'home helps' and the community mental handicap teams. Thirty-four (20.5%) were in open or sheltered employment, four were having work experience, and seven were at college; 60 (36.1%) attended an SEC or an ATC, but 44 (26.5%) had no specific day-time activity (Table 10.1).

These people tended to be older than those living in foster homes or those in residential schools (Figure 10.1).

None of the people who lived independently was profoundly handicapped (Table 10.2); only one was recorded as having 'severe mental retardation'. As would be expected, most of those who lived independently were fully continent (93.0%). Where there were problems of continence, it was occasional night-time incontinence. Ninety-six per cent were fully mobile. There are three people who had little or no useful vision, and a further 22 whose vision was poor even with spectacles. One was deaf, and a further eight had poor hearing. All who lived independently could speak, and most were considered to have good understanding. There was a high level of literacy among the group (Table 10.3), which was not unexpected for people who were able to lead relatively independent lives. Table 10.4 reinforces the picture of a group able to care for themselves reasonably well.

Eighty-nine per cent did not have any severe behavioural problems. Of those who did have behavioural problems, noise and attention-seeking were most frequent, and even the most frequent problem – 'severe noise' – was only noted in eight people.

People with mental handicaps who lived independent or semi-independent lives were the most able of the people on the registers. This was reflected in their range of abilities as well as in their lack of disabilities. However, it is important to recognize that most of them were only able to sustain their 'independence' with a network of support from the statutory and voluntary services.

Group homes may be run by a variety of different agencies. They usually have a small staff, and some do not have any staff living in at night. Some provide permanent homes for a slightly less able group than those who are independent; others are designed to be a stepping-stone for people who will eventually move to an 'independent' life in the community.

The 156 people who lived in group homes were also older than those in foster homes or residential schools (Figure 10.1). Their day-time activity reflected their higher ability than the generality of people with mental handicaps (Table 10.1) – 30 (21.7%) were in open or sheltered employment, a further two were on 'work experience', and nine were at college; 70 (50.7%) attended SECs and ATCs; 21 (15.2%) had no day-time occupation.

The majority (59.4%) were described as mildly or moderately mentally retarded. Seven were recorded as having severe mental retardation, and 27 (17.4%) as 'using mental handicap services' (Table 10.2).

Virtually all the people living in group homes were continent, only one had a frequent problem, and a further four had occasional incontinence; 98.6% of people in group homes were fully mobile; one could not manage stairs, and one could not walk at all without help.

Twenty-four people had poor vision even though they used spectacles. Four were deaf; a further 11 had hearing problems. One person was unable to speak at all, and nine had only basic speech. One person was recorded as having no understanding and six people's understanding was thought to be at a basic level.

The percentage with some degree of literacy, while not being the same as those living independently, was high (Table 10.3). Their level of self-help skills matched those living independently (Table 10.4).

Fourteen people (9%) were described as having a severe behavioural problem. The most frequently recorded were 'withdrawn behaviour' (eight people) and 'attention-seeking' (five people).

Group homes took able individuals who in time might have managed to move into independent accommodation. Some, however, might have needed the additional support provided by professional staff for the rest of their lives.

The residents recorded under 'Other' (96 people) formed a miscellany of residential accommodation that did not fit under any other heading. It included old people's homes, part III accommodation, residences for the physically handicapped, church army hostels, etc. Although not specified in the records, there are indications that some specialist units (e.g. for autism) might have been included in this category.

Summary

This chapter covered people living in residential accommodation not discussed elsewhere in this report.

People in foster homes had characteristics that were similar to those who lived in their family homes. It seems that foster parents will take on the whole range of disability if properly supported. The availability of this sort of care is limited in inner-city areas where space is at a premium. Foster care also has the same time limitations that family care does – namely, that the time an individual can be cared for in this way is limited by the health and survival of the principal foster parent.

Residential schools appeared to accept many young people with behavioural problems; nearly half (42%) of the pupils had one or more severe behavioural problems recorded.

Although the group who lived independently were the most able of all we looked at, their survival within the community depended on a network of daily or weekly support, which may need to be increased particularly in times of crisis or illness.

Most of those in group homes were on the border line of being able to manage independently, but their support needs were greater than those who did live independently. The category 'Other' was a residual catch-all for which no detailed analysis was attempted.

11

Causal diagnosis

Introduction

In the earlier chapters, the abilities and disabilities of people with mental handicaps who were living in different environments has been considered in some detail. It was clear that, because of the close association between physical handicap, behavioural problems and mental handicap, the optimum living environment is determined by factors other than the intellectual deficit. Thus, the underlying cause of the primary intellectual deficit is a relatively unimportant factor when considering strategies to improve the quality of an individual's life. However, an appreciation of cause is of value in another context: if the cause of the problem is understood, then it may be possible to devise rational preventive strategies and to evaluate their effectiveness. In this chapter the available data on causal diagnosis are considered.

Although the registration form included a specific question on causal diagnosis, only limited information was available. Some information was recorded for 3191 (55%) individuals. In many cases it was simply a reiteration of the fact that an individual was intellectually handicapped, for example, they were recorded as having 'profound mental handicap' or 'mild mental handicap'. It is not difficult to understand the reasons for the inadequacy of information in this particular section of the form. Most of the people responsible for completing the registration forms were more interested in the day-to-day care of the affected individuals. For some of the older people, the cause of the handicap had long been forgotten because it had become irrelevant to management. In others, no cause had ever been established. The limited data that were available gave some insights.

Main causes recorded

After excluding vague and ill-defined medical terms, statements of the fact that an individual is mentally handicapped, and diseases that complicate management rather than cause the handicap, the causes of the primary intellectual handicap can be divided into three main groups: autism; chromosomal abnormalities; and diseases of the nervous system.

Chromosomal abnormalities, including Down's syndrome

Roughly one third (975) of those for whom diagnostic information was available had Down's syndrome. This finding is in line with those from other epidemiological investigations (McGrother and Marshall, 1990). A further 24 individuals were affected with other chromosmal abnormalities. The Down's syndrome group were younger than the non-Down's syndrome group (Table 11.1). Their youth might have been the result of either poor survival or a recent increase in incidence.

Table 11.1 Age distribution of people with Down's syndrome compared with all people with all other causes of mental handicaps

Age group	Percentages with Down's syndrome	All other causes of mental handicaps
15–24 years	27.38	24.09
25–34	30.15	26.81
35–44	23.28	17.39
45–54	13.03	11.98
55–65	4.92	9.32
> 65	1.23	10.41

le with Down's syndrome are prone to severe
tory and other infections. They have a high incidence
ui congenital abnormalities, including congenital heart disease.
In the past, most of these conditions were associated with a
high mortality at all ages, though it was most marked in infancy
and adolescence. However, the availability and use of effective treatments has greatly increased life expectancy. It is
unlikely that the incidence of Down's syndrome has increased
significantly during the past 25 years.

The close association between maternal age and Down's
syndrome would lead one to expect that there would only be
a natural increase in the prevalence of the condition if there
were to be a significant upward shift in maternal age in the
absence of selective abortion. The numbers of cases found in
this investigation, which focuses on people over the age of
15 years, are unlikely to have been affected by the policy of
selective amniocentesis and elective abortion, as it was not
introduced until the early 1970s. Therefore, a change in survival patterns is the most likely explanation for the age distribution of the group investigated.

About half of those who had Down's syndrome lived in their
family home (Figure 11.1); a relatively low proportion (14%)
resided in hospital. The degree of mental handicap among
those with Down's syndrome was similar to that of all those
registered – 2.4% were profoundly mentally handicapped, and
29.0% were severely handicapped.

The prevalence of severe physical disability among the
people with Down's syndrome was less than that of the whole
population with mental handicaps (Figure 11.2). They tended
to have fewer severe behavioural problems. These observations are consistent with the well-documented characteristic
of a high degree of empathy among people with Down's syndrome (Buckley and Sacks, 1987).

There is a well-known association between Down's syndrome and maternal age. Although the age of the mother at
the time of the birth was not recorded in the data set, the age
of the 'principal carer' of people living with their families was
recorded. In the vast majority of cases, the principal carer was
the biological mother of the handicapped individual. The age
distribution of the principal carers (a reasonable proxy for the

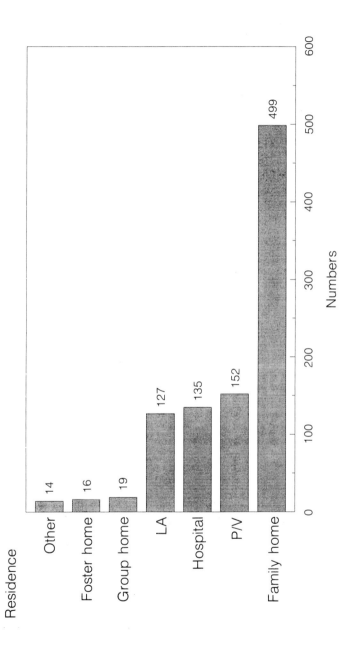

Figure 11.1 Down's syndrome – place of residence.

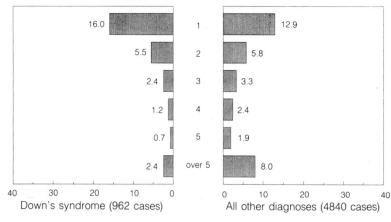

% with Severe Physical Disability Scores

71.1% of people with Down's syndrome and 65.7% of all others have no severe physical disabilities.

Figure 11.2 Down's syndrome (ICD 9 Chapter 14) – percentage with severe physical disability scores.

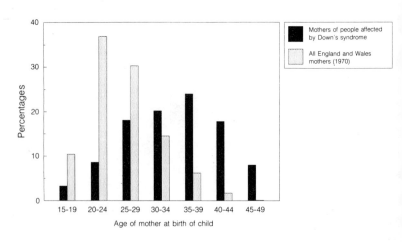

Figure 11.3 Down's syndrome (ICD 9 Chapter 14) – age of mother at birth.

120

mothers) is compared with that of all women in England and
Wales at the time that their babies were born in Figure 11.3.
The 'mothers' of people with Down's syndrome were
significantly older than all mothers. The numbers from which
Figure 11.3 was derived underestimates the skewness of maternal age because the older individuals with Down's syndrome
will have been in residential care, and therefore the age of the
principal carer would not have been recorded.

Diseases of the nervous system

The cause of the mental handicap in 382 cases was said to be
a 'disease of the nervous system'; this broad group included
spina bifida.

One-hundred-and-forty-five had cerebral palsy (Table 11.2).
'Cerebral palsy' is not strictly a cause of mental handicap –
it is a syndrome closely associated with mental handicap, both
of them being due to brain damage at birth. The numbers of
individuals in this category should be regarded as a minimum
estimate of the impact of brain damage on the prevalence of
mental handicaps, since it excludes children who suffered brain
damage without having any motor disability.

Thirty-two had spina bifida. Spina bifida is not a 'cause'
of mental handicap, and a large proportion of people so
affected have normal intelligence. However, the underlying
pathology – a neural tube defect – is associated with

Table 11.2 Diseases of the nervous system and sense organs by age

Disease	15–24	25–34	35–44	45–54	55–64	>65	Total
Bacterial meningitis	1	3	3	0	0	0	7
Other meningitis	5	6	5	4	1	3	24
Encephalitis	3	6	7	0	2	0	18
Intracranial abscess	3	3	2	1	1	2	13
Cerebral degen.	5	3	3	1	1	3	16
Spinocerebellar dis.	1	2	3	0	1	0	8
Cerebral palsy	55	39	26	12	11	2	145
Epilepsy	14	10	11	4	4	3	46
Other	31	24	9	6	4	1	73
Total	118	96	69	28	25	14	350

hydrocephalus, which can be a cause of mental handicap. Spina bifida is often associated with severe physical disabilities.

Meningitis accounted for less than 1% of cases for whom there was a causal diagnosis.

The individuals affected by diseases of the nervous system tended to be younger than the whole group of people with mental handicaps (Figure 11.4). This might be the result of decreased survival in childhood, or a recent increased incidence resulting from improved survival in the perinatal period. This could have been a result of developments in intensive neonatal care. From the available data, it was impossible to establish which of these was the case. People in this group were the most severely mentally handicapped among all of the diagnostic categories (Figure 11.5). As a group they were more severely physically disabled than the generality of people with mental handicaps (Figure 11.6). They did not differ from all with mental handicaps in the prevalence of severe behavioural problems (Figure 11.7).

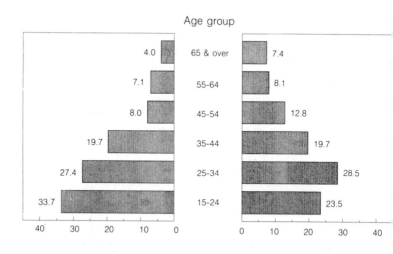

Age group

Diseases of the nervous system (350 cases)   All other diagnoses (5452 cases)

Figure 11.4 Diseases of the nervous system and sense organs – age distribution compared with all others (percentages in each group).

Degree of handicap (% in each group)

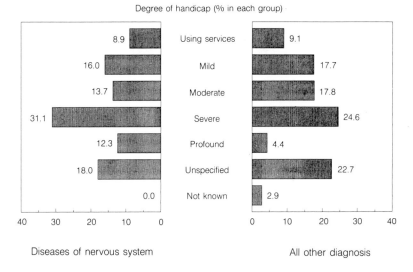

Diseases of nervous system

All other diagnosis

Figure 11.5 Diseases of the nervous system and sense organs – degree of handicap compared with those for all other cases.

Physical disability scores (% in each group)

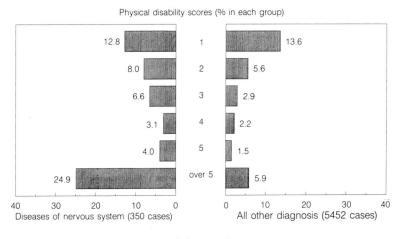

Diseases of nervous system (350 cases)

All other diagnosis (5452 cases)

40.5% of people with diseases of the nervous system and 68.4% of all others have no severe physical disabilities.

Figure 11.6 Diseases of the nervous system and sense organs – severe physical disability scores compared with those for all other cases.

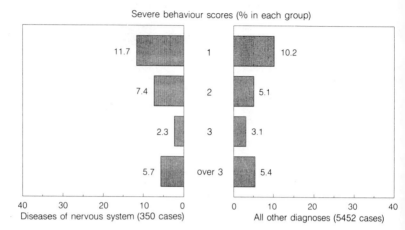

Severe behaviour scores (% in each group)

	Diseases of nervous system (350 cases)		All other diagnoses (5452 cases)
1	11.7		10.2
2	7.4		5.1
3	2.3		3.1
over 3	5.7		5.4

72.9% of people with diseases of the nervous
system and 76.1% of all others have no severe
behavioural problems

Figure 11.7 Diseases of the nervous system and sense organs – severe behaviour scores compared with those for all other cases.

Autism

In 124 cases the underlying explanatory diagnosis was autism. All the people so diagnosed were young (Table 11.3). Their relative youth was unlikely to have been the result of either a real increase in incidence rates, or low survival rates of affected individuals; it is more likely to have been attributable to a change in diagnostic practices.

Autism has only been recognized as a distinct clinical entity relatively recently (Kanner, 1943). Before 1943, affected individuals would either have been assigned to another diagnostic category or no cause for the handicap would have been established. Clearly, very few people had their causal diagnosis revised following the identification of autism as a syndrome. This may have been either because a change in 'diagnosis' would have made no difference to their management, or because diagnosis of autism is difficult after a particular age.

124

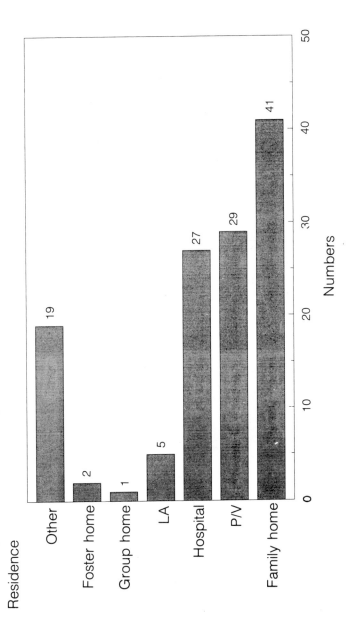

Figure 11.8 Autism – place of residence.

Table 11.3 Distribution of people with autism compared with all others with mental handicaps according to age (percentage)

Age group	Autism	All with mental handicap
15–24 years	38.71	24.06
25–34	44.35	28.34
35–44	14.52	19.63
45–54	2.42	12.51
55–64	0.00	7.98
> 64	0.00	7.14
All	100.00	100.00

Despite their youth, a smaller proportion of people with autism lived in their family homes than would have been expected (Figure 11.8). A relatively high proportion lived in hospital. The differences in place of residence are likely to reflect the behavioural problems that characterize autism.

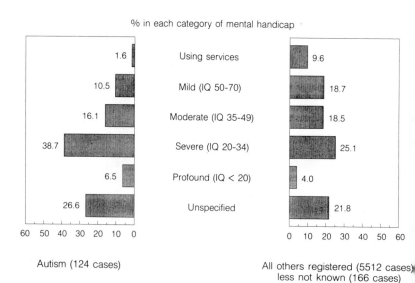

% in each category of mental handicap

	Autism		All others
Using services	1.6		9.6
Mild (IQ 50-70)	10.5		18.7
Moderate (IQ 35-49)	16.1		18.5
Severe (IQ 20-34)	38.7		25.1
Profound (IQ < 20)	6.5		4.0
Unspecified	26.6		21.8

Autism (124 cases)

All others registered (5512 cases) less not known (166 cases)

Figure 11.9 Autism and degree of mental handicap.

% with severe behaviour scores

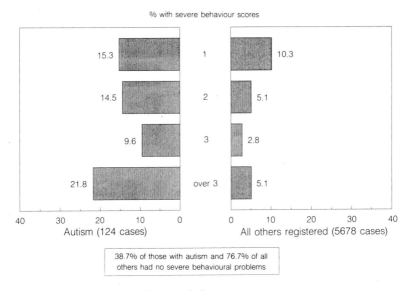

Figure 11.10 Autism and severe behaviour scores.

% with severe physical disability scores

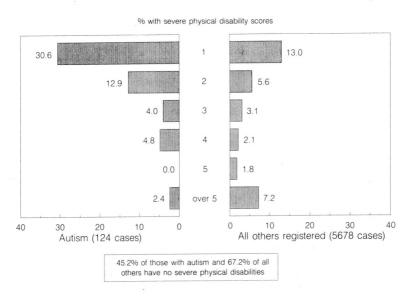

Figure 11.11 Autism and severe physical disability scores.

127

A high proportion of the people with autism were classified as either 'Severely' or 'Profoundly' mentally handicapped – 45.3% compared with 29.1% of all the people on the registers (Figure 11.9). The proportion with one or more severe behavioural problems was high (Fig 11.10), and the group scored at a relatively high level on the 'Severe' physical disability scales (Fig 11.11).

Mental illness and mental handicap

The issue of mental illness among peple with mental handicaps is complex. The only 'psychiatric' syndrome that is consistently associated with mental handicap is infantile autism. However, people with mental handicaps do suffer from mental illness, and their mental illnesses complicate management. The

Table 11.4 Psychiatric diagnoses among people with mental handicaps

		Age group			
ICD code	Disease	15–44	45–64	> 64	Total
290	Senile and presenile organic psychoses	0	3	4	7
291	Alcoholic psychoses	0	0	1	1
294	Other organic psychotic conditions	1	3	0	4
295	Schizophrenic psychoses	85	55	22	162
296	Affective psychoses	8	15	2	25
297	Paranoid states	1	0	0	1
298	Other non-organic psychoses	39	10	10	59
299	Psychoses with origin in childhood	153	5	0	158
300	Neurotic disorders	28	12	1	41
301	Personality disorders	19	19	2	40
302	Sexual deviations and disorders	1	2	0	3
307	Special signs and symptoms	6	0	0	6
310	Non-psychotic after brain damage	3	1	2	6
311	Depressive disorders NEC	8	9	3	20
312	Disturbances of conduct	14	5	2	21
313	Disturbances of emotion	10	2	1	13
All		376	141	50	567

diagnosis section on the registration form was inconsistently used by the people who made the assessments, and, although it provides some information on mental illness, the data must be taken as providing a minimum estimate of the impact of mental illness among people with mental handicaps.

The files were searched for any entry that referred to mental illness (ICD 9 Chapter 5) within any of the diagnostic fields. Five-hundred-and-sixty-seven cases (17.8% of all for whom diagnostic data were available) had been diagnosed as having some form of mental illness (Table 11.4). The diagnostic categories with the largest number of cases were schizophrenic psychoses (ICD 295) and psychoses with origin in childhood (ICD 299). The ICD category 'schizophrenic psychoses' includes simple schizophrenia, hebephrenic schizophrenia, catatonic schizophrenia, acute schizophrenic episode, residual schizophrenia and some other ill-defined psychotic disorders. It excludes infantile autism and childhood schizophrenia, both of which are included in the category 'psychoses with origin in childhood'. It is possible that some of the adult individuals whose mental handicap was in fact due to infantile autism may have been misclassified within the schizophrenic psychoses.

About half of those who had been diagnosed as having a 'schizophrenic psychosis' were aged over 45 years. Clearly the fact that at least 5% of those with mental handicap were affected with this group of disorders represents a problem that must be taken into account when planning services (Ineichen, 1984; Williams, 1971).

12

Severity of disability

Introduction

People with mental handicaps are a diverse group. Clear differences emerged between the characteristics of people in different residential settings. In an attempt to discover whether people with similar levels of disability are clustered together, in this chapter, people with mental handicaps have been divided into four broad categories on the basis of their physical and behavioural problems.

The basis of the categorization

The disabilities and problems of each registered individual was rated in the course of their regular assessment. The broad areas covered were as follows:

- Physical problems
  - night urinary/faecal continence
  - day urinary/faecal continence
  - ability to walk, feed, wash, dress
- Sensory and communication problems
  - vision
  - hearing
  - use of speech

- Behavioural problems
  - hitting and attacking others (personal aggression)
  - damaging clothing or furniture
  - excessive activity (pacing, disturbed nights)
  - attention-seeking
  - self-injury (head banging, picking)
  - delinquent acts (pilfering, fire-raising)
  - unacceptable personal habits (masturbation in public, spitting)
  - wandering off
  - noise (screaming, shouting, verbal aggression)
  - negative, withdrawn, or unco-operative

Each of the indices had been rated on a scale of either three or five points. An individual 'scored' one point for each item that represented a problem, irrespective of its frequency or severity.

On the above basis, the minimum score on the rating scale was 0 and the maximum was 21. The higher scores indicate greater levels of disability.

The individuals aged over 15 years of age on the registers were divided into four groups of roughly equal size according to their scores on the above 'rating scale'. These groups are compared and contrasted in this chapter. The definition and sizes of the groups were as follows:

- Score 0–1 – 26% of cases (Type One)
- Score 2–4 – 25% of cases (Type Two)
- Score 5–9 – 24% of cases (Type Three)
- Score 10 and over – 25% of cases (Type Four)

Severity of disability and degree of mental handicap

The degree of mental handicap had been assessed in 3782 individuals, about three-quarters of all cases. The assessment was often the opinion of the keyworker involved rather than a formal measurement of the IQ, or the 'mental age'. The categories that were used were those defined in the International Classification of Diseases (ICD) 9th edition, and were as follows:

- Profound mental retardation – IQ < 20
- Severe mental retardation – IQ 20–34
- Moderate mental retardation – IQ 35–49
- Mild mental retardation – IQ 50–70
- Unspecified mental retardation

A further category, 'Using services', was introduced to cover people who used the services designed for people with mental handicaps but were considered to have an IQ of above 70. It is believed this latter category was used instead of 'Unspecified Mental Handicap' by some of the people making assessments.

Table 12.1 shows the distribution of the people according to their 'severity type' and their degree of mental handicap, where specified. There was only one profoundly handicapped person among the Type One individuals (those least handicapped). The majority (74.4%) of the Type One people were assessed as either moderately or mildly mentally handicapped. By contrast, over 80% of those of Type Four were either severely or profoundly mentally handicapped; 85% of the 237 individuals who were profoundly handicapped fell into Type Four, the most severely affected with concurrent physical, sensory and behavioural problems; 3.9% of those with a mild mental handicap were in Type Four. The most obvious explanation for these findings is that severe and profound mental handicap is closely associated with brain damage at birth – brain damage is also associated with disorders of autonomic, sensory and motor function.

Table 12.1 Disability type and degree of mental handicap

| | Disability type | | | |
Degree of mental handicap	One	Two	Three	Four
Using services	158	101	65	46
Mild	436	308	151	44
Moderate	265	331	242	104
Severe	82	217	396	599
Profound	1	5	30	201
Total known	942	962	884	994

The close correlation between the implied IQ and the numbers of associated physical, sensory, and behavioural problems is interesting; it might be taken to indicate that IQ has a utility. It would be wrong to use IQ as the sole indicator, or predictor, of the severity of the associated problems and disabilities of an individual, but perhaps it would be equally wrong to ignore it.

Severity of disability and epilepsy

The proportion of individuals in each of the severity groups who were affected with epilepsy and the degree of control achieved are shown in Figure 12.1. The proportion with epilepsy increased in frequency with behaviour, sensory, and physical disability scores. The difference between Types One and Two and between Types Two and Three was less marked than the difference between Type Four and the other groups. Whereas about 10% of Type One individuals were affected, up to 30% of Type Four individuals were affected. Among the Types One and Two individuals with epilepsy, most were controlled. Nearly all those with uncontrolled epilepsy were in Types Three and Four.

There is a general tendency for the proportion affected with epilepsy to decrease with increasing age; in particular there are no people with uncontrolled epilepsy among those over 55 years of age. It is likely this is due to differential survival.

There was insufficient data to establish whether there was a common cause of the epilepsy and the sensory and physical disabilities, or whether the associated disabilities, including problems with behaviour, were the result of the uncontrolled, or uncontrollable, epilepsy.

Severity of disability and place of residence

About half of the Type One individuals were resident in their own homes; 10.5% lived in hospitals; and just over 20% were living in either LA or P/V accommodation (Table 12.2). One-third of the Type Four individuals – those with the greatest concurrent disabilities – lived in their family homes, and 47%

Severity of disability

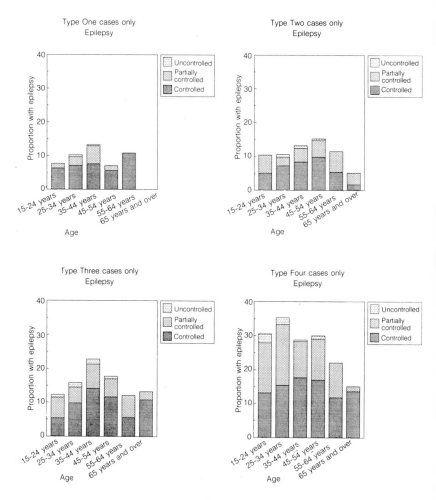

Figure 12.1 Proportion affected with epilepsy and degree of control.

lived in hospitals. It is not surprising that such a high proportion of the severely affected individuals lived in hospital, as they would have required more intensive attention and would be unlikely to fit into the type of accommodation provided in the community. However, the strikingly large proportion of the severely disabled who live at home is likely to

134

Table 12.2 Disability type and place of residence, ( ) = column percentages

Place of residence	Disability type			
	One	*Two*	*Three*	*Four*
Family home or school	609 (49.1)	546 (45.0)	482 (41.3)	389 (32.4)
LA homes	118 (9.5)	155 (12.8)	78 (6.7)	84 (6.9)
P/V homes	147 (11.8)	152 (12.5)	98 (8.4)	111 (9.2)
Hospitals	130 (10.5)	265 (21.8)	463 (39.6)	562 (46.8)
Other	210 (16.9)	112 (9.2)	47 (4.0)	55 (4.6)
Total	1241 (100)	1214 (100)	1168 (100)	1201 (100)

reflect the inadequacy of provision of alternatives to the hospital.

The category 'Other' accommodation included people who lived independently, those in group homes, foster homes, and NHS hostels. About half of the people of Type One who lived in 'Other' accommodation were in fact living independently. By contrast, the substantial majority of the Type Four individuals who were in 'Other' accommodation were living in specialist NHS hostels – most of which were on the campuses of the long-stay mental handicap hospitals.

The ages of all the carers was not known, but there is no reason to suppose that the 67% for whom the age was available differed from those for whom it was not. Sixteen per cent of the Type Four individuals, and 22% of the Type Three individuals were being cared for by a parent who was over 65 years of age (Table 12.3).

Table 12.3 Disability type and age of carer (residents in family home)

	Disability type			
Age of carer	One	Two	Three	Four
< 45 years	27	40	38	54
45–64 years	191	211	169	183
> 65 years	198	142	67	46

Summary

There is clear evidence for an association between behavioural problems and physical disability and the degree of mental handicap. The association is not perfect, and it is therefore unsafe to abandon either measure. The severity of physical and behavioural problems correlates closely with the prevalence of epilepsy and the level of control achieved. About one-quarter of the people with mental handicaps over the age of 15 years within the NW Thames region were severely disabled, and because of concurrent epilepsy would present serious management difficulties. Some of these people were living at home in the care of their ageing parents. It appeared there was no alternative to this arrangement at the time.

13

Discussion

Introduction

People with mental handicaps are some of the most vulnerable in our society. Few of them will be able to live their lives without considerable support from parents, professionally trained carers and the community as a whole. The services required to give them the necessary support should not simply be left to evolve – they need planning and financing within a suitable organizational structure. The nature of the people affected by mental handicaps is such that they themselves are unable to develop schemes for care and raise the level of public commitment.

In most countries where services are well developed, there is a history of committed individuals with a personal interest in the welfare of people with mental handicaps pressurizing the authorities to provide and improve services. However, in some countries the level and type of provision is determined by tradition, fashion, and ideology, with little or no understanding of the complexities of the problems faced by people with mental handicaps, their families, and the communities into which they are born.

The data presented in this book reveal that people with mental handicaps are a diverse group. The importance, and sometimes the dominance, of associated handicaps may be lost within simplistic formulations such as 'mental handicap', 'people with learning difficulties', or 'mental retardation'. The data has identified significant unmet needs, inappropriate provision, unrealistic plans, and a heavy reliance on families. There is a clear need for regular, objective information in order to plan and evaluate services for people with mental handicaps.

Background to the registers

The KCW health authority set up the first register of people with mental handicaps in the NW Thames region. Its development began in the late 1970s, and its initial aims were limited. It was designed to maintain up-to-date records of individuals with mental handicaps, where they lived, and the level of their abilities and disabilities. Its purpose was to facilitate service developments. Over the years, the amount and type of information collected (and systematically updated) on each person has been modified in response to the needs of the providers of care. From its early stages, the register has been used by a wide range of individuals and agencies. Its perceived value increased with usage. In the early 1980s, the RHA decided that it would be advantageous for each of its districts to have and to use the same system as KCW's. In order to speed up developments, specific monies were made available to each district for the purchase of hardware and software and to supplement staff salaries. Some districts established a register rapidly and maintained it for many years. Others made a slow start and never achieved useful and comprehensive systems.

The reasons that some districts succeeded and others did not was not investigated by the authorities, but informal enquiries indicated that a number of factors were relevant.

The success of information systems depends first on obtaining the original data, and second, ensuring that it is kept up to date. In order to collect and update the data required for a register, it is essential to liaise with the large number of individuals and organizations concerned with the day-to-day care of people with mental handicaps. The identification of these and the establishment of good working relationships depends to a great extent upon the personality, maturity, and drive of those appointed to manage the registers. Some authorities were able to recruit and retain highly motivated and experienced people, while others were not. The register staff who encouraged people to use the database they had helped to create and maintain tended to do better.

The success of the registers was also affected by the attitude of management. Some managers saw the register system as an essential planning and managerial tool. Districts in which this attitude prevailed produced more comprehensive and up-to-date information. By contrast, some local managers regarded the collection of information as a fringe activity not directly related to the day-to-day problems of providing a service. Districts in which such management attitudes prevailed did not produce good-quality data.

Since 1984 there have been a number of managerial and structural changes in the NHS and in the social services. In addition, for the past few years there have been uncertainties regarding which agencies will have long-term and lead responsibility for the care of people with mental handicaps. Proposals to transfer responsibility from the NHS to the LA social service departments were announced some time ago, and formal plans have only recently been published. Clearly, changes and uncertainty affect morale. There is some indication that not all of the current NHS managers have the necessary interest and commitment to the problems to enable financing of the registers to continue.

This analysis of detailed data on people with mental handicaps in the region presented in this book is the first to have been attempted. It is likely to be the last for a long time since less than half of the registers that provided data for this exercise are being maintained, and the future of the others is in serious doubt.

Prevalence of mental handicap

None of the registers consistently registered people under the age of 15 years. Some had a policy of not registering children under certain ages, even though they were known to have mental handicaps. Clearly, the regional data set yielded poor-quality data about people in the younger age groups.

A mathematical model using the data on adults and adolescents indicates there are about 14 000 people of all ages (4.04 per 1000 total population) with mental handicaps who either live in or originated from the NW Thames region. All of these people, and some of their families, will need care, access to special facilities, and support for the whole of their lives.

Estimates of the prevalence of mental handicap are affected by the varying definitions used, the different professional perspectives of those working in the field, and the absence of a consensus about the tools used for assessment – including a reluctance to use properly standardized instruments. Taking account of differences in definition, the estimate of the prevalence of people with mental handicaps from this investigation is in line with other estimates.

From the limited data that are available, there is no evidence to suggest that the number of people affected with mental handicaps is decreasing. In recent years, a high proportion of pregnant women over the age of 35 have been screened for the presence of foetuses affected with chromosomal abnormalities or other untreatable conditions with a view to elective termination. This policy has undoubtedly reduced the incidence of births of affected babies to older women. However, babies with chromosomal abnormalities, including Down's syndrome, continue to be conceived by and born to younger women. However, recent developments in screening technology will almost certainly make such tests available to all women.

Over the past half century, improvements in ante- and intranatal care have made a significant contribution to the prevention of damage to normal foetuses and the newborn. On the one hand, this has reduced the numbers of babies with congenital infections, and those affected by adverse pregnancies. On the other hand, modern treatments have increased the survival rate of vulnerable babies who have a high probability of mental handicap, and who in the past would have died shortly after birth. The intensive postnatal care of extreme premature babies is a good example.

Medical care after the immediate postnatal period has also had its impact on the prevalence of people with mental handicaps. The ease with which infections can now be treated has reduced mortality throughout life. Surgical and medical treatments of the physical malformations and diseases, from which many people with mental handicaps suffer, is now much more effective, widely available, and increasingly utilized. General improvements in living conditions – including diet and the standard of accommodation – has also resulted in people living longer, including those with mental handicaps. The net result is that although there may have been some reduction in incidence, this has been counteracted by increased survival. Thus, like the general population, the population of people with mental handicaps is ageing.

Down's syndrome provides an excellent example of the impact of these developments. In the immediate postwar period, many children born with Down's syndrome had died by their early 20s; currently they are surviving to their 50s and beyond. The full impact of the developments in medical care have yet to be felt. It is likely the prevalence of affected individuals will increase, even if the incidence rate decreases or is maintained at its present level. Moreover, an increasing number of affected individuals will survive to have the additional problems associated with old age, such as dementia and cancers.

Measurement of intelligence

The unifying characteristics of the people discussed in this book is their intellectual impairment. Over the last century, the understanding of intellectual function has changed. It used to be thought of as a fixed biological attribute, which led to the practice of classifying children at an early age and certifying them as mentally retarded, with a view to them spending their lives in special institutions. It is now apparent that intellectual functioning is the result of a number of highly interactive processes: it can be affected both beneficially and adversely by the social environment, educational practices, and by con-current physical and sensory disabilities.

Although the notion of IQ has been abandoned by some professional workers, the concept of an individual having a more or less precisely measurable level of 'intelligence' still underlies the subclassification of 'mental retardation' within the International Classification of Diseases and Causes of Death (ICD). 'Mild Mental Retardation' is used to designate people with IQ levels between 50–70; 'Moderate' for people with levels between 35–59; 'Severe' between 20–34; while those with an IQ level under 20 are designated as having a 'Profound Mental Retardation'. Today, in many care situations an individual's degree of mental handicap is estimated without recourse to formal intelligence testing; indeed, in this investigation it was found that only a minority of the people had had a formal intelligence test. Analyses of the data reveals that the informally assessed 'degree of mental handicap' appears to correlate with certain abilities and disabilities (reading, writing, counting, and so on), with the general level of support that individuals can be expected to require, and with the type of accommodation in which they live. In view of these observations, it is reasonable to ask why there is a reluctance to make measurements of IQ and use them appropriately in conjunction with other assessment data.

As the intellectual attainment of an individual is not solely determined by a fixed and measurable biological characteristic, the use of IQ as the sole basis or classification would be damaging to the best interests of the individual. However, there are important distinctions between those people categorized as having 'Mild Mental Handicap' and those with 'Severe Mental Handicap', which includes 'Moderate', 'Severe', and 'Profound'. Virtually all in the latter group have some degree of brain damage, and this is nearly always associated with physical disabilities, in addition to the intellectual impairment. Those affected in this way will be dependent upon other people for the basic elements of their existence throughout their lives.

Multiple handicap

Although the primary disability of the subjects of this book is an intellectual impairment, no single term describes them satisfactorily. Virtually all have difficulties with reading, writing, and counting, which places severe restrictions on the conduct of their everyday lives. These difficulties are usually coupled with problems in understanding the meaning of many of the transactions taken for granted by most people. Many people with mental handicaps have additional physical handicaps which can cause problems with mobility, continence, feeding, dressing, and washing. A significant proportion behave in ways that are not generally acceptable. Although some problems with behaviour may be exacerbated by environmental factors, there is no evidence to show that all 'behavioural problems' can be completely controlled.

People with mental handicaps form a group united by their intellectual impairment but divided by their physical, behavioural, social, and other handicaps. These individual differences are of enormous practical importance for service planning. Because of the variety and complexity of their handicaps, it is unlikely that their needs will be met satisfactorily within a single model of care. Some may thrive in sheltered accommodation integrated with a local community and supported by well-organized day-care facilities; while others may be able to cope with a semi-independent life, provided there is someone to whom they can turn in times of need; yet others may require expert care and attention throughout the day and night in an environment that is closer to a hospital than to a domestic home.

In the past, plans for the care of people with mental handicaps have tended to be based on fashionable notions and ideological considerations rather than an objective consideration of detailed information about individuals. There have been few attempts to evaluate different types of care for different individuals against realistic expectations of what their optimal quality of life could be.

Impact of current policy

Families

In this investigation, the information available on people aged under 15 years was limited in quantity and of doubtful quality. At an early stage in the analysis, a decision was made to concentrate on people over 15 years of age. The family still cares for the great majority of people with mental handicaps between the ages of 15–25. It is clear that there are now very few children under the age of 15 years permanently resident in hospital. It may be concluded that the vast majority of people up to 25 years are cared for by their families. Even between the ages of 25–35 a substantial proportion are still totally dependent on their families.

The concept of 'normalization' defined by Bank-Mikkelsen (1969) and popularized by Wolfensberger (1972) in the US was based on the notion that people with mental handicaps had a right to live a 'normal' life in ordinary houses within their own communities. The idea was incorporated into planning philosophy in the mid-1960s. The initial impact on service planning was the adoption of a policy designed to close the hospitals that had been the mainstay of care for the previous 60 or so years. The contraction of the large hospitals has not been accompanied by significant building of alternative accommodation, consequentially, a greater burden of care has had to be taken by parents.

There are now large numbers of people with mental handicaps, both children and adults, who live at home. Their parents are ageing. In general, they remain at home until one of their parents dies or becomes too ill to provide care. At that stage emergency admission to some sort of institution becomes necessary. This investigation provided no data on either the physical or mental health of the parents, and to our knowledge such data are not routinely collected and considered by the authorities responsible for planning and providing care.

The crudest measure of the time limit that an individual can be cared for at home by his or her family is the length of time that the principal carer – normally the mother – is likely to survive. It is estimated that in the NW Thames region, 50 people with mental handicaps will need to be found accommodation each year during the next decade. This estimate does not include essential admissions for other reasons, and assumes that the life expectancy of women occupied in caring for mentally and physically handicapped adults is the same as that of women in general. There is no basis for that assumption, and we feel it may be unrealistically optimistic.

The desirability of a system whereby parents are expected to be the fulcrum of care for a significant number of people until their own death is questionable. In many cases – both for the sake of the parents and for the person who is handicapped – it may be preferable for the handicapped person to leave the family home at an earlier age. Indeed, in 'normal' families the children leave home to establish their own lives in their early 20s.

It is important that each responsible authority monitors the ages and health of parents. They should be able to offer long-term care placements at intervals, with the option of short visits at first to help acceptance. At the very least this would ensure that in a crisis, people with mental handicaps would go to places that they know and where they are known. It should help to minimize the trauma of sudden ruptures of personal relationships, the introduction to a new and strange environment, and unfamiliar patterns of life. In the longer term there is a need to reconsider the acceptability of a system of care that is substantially dependent upon parents committing their lives to the total care of their offspring.

The difficulties with the present arrangements are compounded by many people with mental handicaps requiring regular expert medical and other attention because of their concurrent long-term illnesses and disabilities. In line with the policy of 'normalization', there has been a move towards integrating the medical and paramedical care for this group with that for the general population.

The belief is that this policy will decrease the possibility of the handicapped person being stigmatized, however, it has its disadvantages. The mother of a child with Down's syndrome who has problems with hearing and sight, has congenital heart disease, and difficulties with mobility may find herself spending a great deal of time attending a variety of specialist outpatient departments. The 'child' may disrupt the clinic and embarrass the mother, and even if he or she does not, the regular clinic visits will tend to disrupt her life and that of the rest of her family. In view of the increasing reliance on families to provide care, consideration should be given to the reintroduction of integrated clinics for people with multiple handicaps.

Hospitals

Of the current residents in the region's hospitals, 1500 will have to be accommodated elsewhere if they are to be closed within the next ten years. The remainder will have died. Many of the current residents have more than one severe physical or behavioural problem; they will be complicated and expensive to settle elsewhere. Their disabilities are more severe and their needs are greater than those of people who are now living in P/V or LA accommodation. Few residential facilities have been developed or planned for multiply handicapped people – many appear to be unrealistically financed. In line with current policy, the hospitals are unwilling to accept admissions. This has effectively closed the door to elective admissions of people from their family homes.

The nature of the hospital population has changed over the past decade. The most able have already been resettled in the community, and as a consequence today's average hospital patient has greater needs and is more dependent than was the case in the past. The resettlement of the most able, who often used to assist in the care of those more disabled, has removed a source of help from the hospitals. This places even greater pressures on the nursing and other staff.

As the process of resettlement continues and the most able are discharged, the cost per resident patient in hospital will continue to increase. In 1979, the cost per resident per year was £13 393, at 1988/9 prices; by 1989 this had risen to £21 159, a rise of 58% over inflation. The costs of the residual hospital population will continue to rise, and some authorities have not taken this into account in their budgeting. The chronic shortage of funds, the ever-present threats of closure at an undisclosed date, and the increasing proportion of patients requiring intensive attention is having an adverse effect on staff morale and functioning in some hospitals.

Concentration on the logistics of re-accommodating those now in hospital tends to understate the full scale of the problems created by the hospital closure programme. There are now people living outside hospitals who need the type of care that is only available in hospitals. The pursuance of a ruthless hospital closure programme is not feasible without the concurrent development of alternatives for those not yet admitted.

It appears that the hospital closure programme may have proceeded at too fast a pace for the authorities to produce appropriate alternative accommodation for those with multiple handicaps. It may be necessary to reconsider current policy and plan to retain some adequately funded facilities in existing hospitals for the mentally handicapped until the necessary infrastructure to care for people with multiple handicaps is established and funded elsewhere. These may be in a different and more homelike type of hospital.

Voluntary organizations

The voluntary organizations were formed as pressure groups to protect the interests of and improve services for people with mental handicaps. They are charities, and depend very much on the commitment of local people, many of whom have personal experience of mental handicap as parents. Most are affiliated to MENCAP.

In the past, the funds voluntary organizations raised were used to provide extra facilities that were outside the scope of the statutory services. More recently, some societies have raised funds to provide local residential accommodation for people for whom hospital admission was inappropriate. In these schemes the monies raised by the societies were used to buy buildings and convert and furnish them. The revenue necessary to pay for staff, maintenance, and consumables was provided by the LAs on the basis of a fixed amount per resident per week. The weekly fees were negotiated annually between each society and its LA. No attempt was made to build in a profit element. In some cases the fees negotiated were unrealistic as they took little account of the capital invested, nor did they take account of the fixed costs that had to be borne by the society even if a place was not occupied. This approach has two important consequences: first, the finances of the societies may be made insecure and great efforts will be required to raise further charitable funds in order to remain solvent; second, the LAs have an unrealistic appreciation of the true cost of care outside hospitals.

The current policy of closing hospitals has increased the demand for residential places in the community. The LAs respond to this new demand in two ways: they can provide the accommodation themselves, or make arrangements with third parties – the voluntary societies or the private sector. Central government encourages the authorities to enable rather than provide and the unrealistic costing of places in the voluntary sector make it an attractive provider. Thus, current policy places the voluntary organizations under pressure to increase the amount and broaden the type of residential provision they provide.

As the voluntary societies begin to accept reponsibility for a larger and more disabled group of people, their character will inevitably change. In order to fulfil their new role they will have to employ a larger number and variety of professional staff. Their financial structures will have to be reconsidered in commercial terms.

The influence of the professional employees and the employees of the client LA may diminish the influence and role of the members, mostly parents. These changes have important implications: they may lessen the commitment of the members; they may result in resignations of committee members who feel devalued; there may be a general deterioration of morale; and the possibility of continued charitable fund-raising will tend to diminish. In some parts of NW Thames this has already begun to happen. In order to avoid further problems, it is essential that managers employed by the statutory authorities develop a more sensitive approach to the societies and their members, recognize the reasons for their existence, and value the knowledge and commitment of their members.

Social services

The social service departments of LAs have provided residential and other care for the least disabled people with mental handicaps for many years. The imposition of a concept of community care by central government, and the transfer of primary responsiblity for the care from the NHS places a heavy burden on the resources of the LAs. Although there is great enthusiasm among the professional staff of the social services departments, it is not universally shared by the elected members and executives of the LAs.

Thus far, the experience of LA social servcies departments has been limited to the provision of services for people with mild or moderate mental handicaps. The residential accommodation, social education centres, staff training, and general philosophy developed by the departments over many years has been directed towards this group of people. People with severe and multiple handicaps present a different series of problems, and time will be required to adjust to new circumstances.

The analysis of the data from the NW Thames region clearly indicates that there are substantial and significant differences between the needs of the people with severe or profound mental handicaps and those with mild and moderate handicaps. In addition to their concurrent physical handicaps and medical problems, the severely and profoundly mentally handicapped may have intractable behavioural problems. Many people require attention throughout the day and night, dietary supervision, regular medication, and other interventions that require specialist skilled manpower. Moreover, the type of building that may be appropriate for the mildly and moderately mentally handicapped is likely to be totally inadequate for those severely affected. It is unreasonable to expect the LAs to build up the necessary network of skills and facilities in a short time – the problems that will be encountered will be greatest in central urban areas where costs are higher and the recruitment and retention of skilled staff is more difficult.

The financial implications of the transfer of responsibility from the NHS to LAs are far-reaching. In the past, the care of people affected with severe mental and multiple handicaps was funded centrally. In the future, monies will come from the funds of LAs. The needs of people with mental handicaps will have to compete with those of the children's service, the elderly, the mentally ill, education, and the many other enterprises that are essential functions of the LAs.

A major result of these policy changes is that there is no guarantee that the needs of people with mental handicaps will be adequately financed, or that funding will be consistent across the country. Although finance in the form of 'dowries' has been transferred to LAs in respect of people resettled from hospitals, no equivalent finance has been made available for those who in the past would have been admitted to hospital. In many areas the dowry payments themselves have proved inadequate and need to be supplemented by monies from other sources. Moreover, there is no protection for the monies originnally designated for people with mental handicaps. Both LAs and health services can use these funds for other services as they see fit. Unless there is a clear national policy for funding care, it is possible that in the future the provision of care will become uneven and parents may be tempted to relocate to areas governed by LAs that maintain a high standard of service.

Day-care services

The provision of day-care facilities is a unique responsibility of the social service departments of LAs. The mainstay of provision are the social education centres (SECs), their predecessors were the adult training centres (ATCs). SECs are normally located in the same building or on the same campus as the special needs centres. Usually they are managed as a single organization. The SECs are designed for the able with mental handicaps, whereas the special needs centres focus on those with multiple disabilities. In order to make use of residential facilities, it is essential that day-care is available – in NW Thames there are some residential places in the community that are not used because day-care is not available.

Current policies have far-reaching effects on the day service. Hospitals provide day-care on site; when patients are discharged their day-care becomes the responsibility of the local social service departments. SECs have had to expand to provide space for the first wave of people discharged from hospital. Many have now become unacceptably large and as a result staff find it difficult to organize with the sort of flexibility and sensitivity that the disparate needs of their students require. Future needs can only be met by increasing the number and variety of centres.

The people remaining in hospital, who are expected to be discharged in the near future, will need day services similar to those available in the special needs units because of their multiple and severe problems. Such facilities are more expensive than the SECs.

The hospital closure policy has another impact on the need for day-care facilities. In the past, many people with mental handicaps would have been admitted to hospital during their adolescence; they now remain with their families. Their need for day-care has been partially met by extending the role of the special schools. These schools now sometimes accept children as young as two years old, and often keep them as pupils until the age of 19 years. After 19 some of the more able have been enrolled in further education colleges, often with great success. There is a limit to the time that this transition can mask the need for an expansion of day-care, and it appears that this limit has now been reached.

No additional funds have been made available to LAs to provide extra day-care facilities. In the NW Thames region, nearly 10% of people age 30–44 who lived in their family homes had no day service; this is an unacceptably high proportion.

Elderly people with mental handicaps also need day-care. In some instances it can be provided within the generic geriatric service, but not all people fit happily into this provision. As the population in the community ages, this will become an increasing problem.

The need for information

People with mental handicaps can be identified early in their life. Their likely needs in the short-, medium-, and long-term can be established. It should be possible to plan services for each individual rather than hope that facilities planned on the basis of crude forecasts and population models will meet their needs. This is one of the few groups of individuals for whom such a sophisticated approach to planning is possible.

Unfortunately, the obvious advantages of developing services on this basis has never been exploited. In order to provide and monitor services for these individuals it is essential to maintain an efficient and accessible information system. Few authorities responsible for the provision of services have made the necessary investment and commitment to such systems.

The need for proper information systems today is greater than ever because the services are increasingly becoming dispersed both geographically and administratively. In the past, most of the people involved in care were employed in mental handicap hospitals in which there was a clearly defined hierarchical employment structure, usually headed by the medical superintendent and matron. Today, even within the hospitals, the extent and limits of the responsibilities of the different professions are not clearly defined; rarely is there a single named professional who has the ultimate responsibility for an individual's care.

Outside the hospitals, a wide range of people are involved in the care of people with mental handicaps: social workers, teachers, community nurses, general practitioners, medical specialists, psychiatrists, instructors, general residential care staff, day-care staff, psychologists, occupational, speech and physiotherapists, together with parents and members of voluntary societies. Although there is usually a community mental handicap team with responsibility to each individual, there is no single professionally qualified person with the ultimate responsibility.

Some of the care services are managed by the health service, others by the LA social services departments, and yet others by non-statutory organizations. The turnover of managers and many of the professional staff is high – sometimes so high that the length of time in a particular post is too short for the incumbent to become fully appraised of the local situation and the life-long problems of those with mental handicaps and their families. In these circumstances, an efficient and effective system of care can only be provided if the people providing care are supported by a proper information system.

The need for information

A good information system will enable the progress of an individual to be monitored over time, and progress to be audited against accepted standards and realistic expectations. It should make it possible to evaluate different interventions and types of residential provisions. The data that were collected and updated within the districts of the NW Thames regions over a number of years gives some insight into the potential of good quality information in this field. Unfortunately, the indications are that many of the registers were incomplete, inadequately updated, and in some districts their purposes are ill understood by key managers. The lack of universal managerial appreciation of the need for and potential use of information systems in this field had led to them being under-funded and unsupported.

A comprehensive information system about people with mental handicaps is achievable with current technology. The maintenance of such a system is not prejudicial to those registered, indeed quite the opposite – it can contribute to the enhancement of their quality of care provided the data are used properly. Much of the information that is essential is sensitive and confidential; access to this type of information about a named person must be limited to professionally trained people with a legitimate interest in the handicapped individual. It is not management information. However, the collated data is essential for planning, and must be accessible to management. Without clear rules and trust between the many people involved in care, no system will succeed. Although most of the registers that supplied the anonymous information used in this investigation are no longer operating, it is hoped that the potential of such systems will be recognized in the future, and that this potential will be exploited.

It is inevitable that people with mental handicaps will continue to consume a significant amount of resources, including money, skilled manpower, accommodation, equipment, and medical services. Clearly, it is important that the use of these resources is well planned and managed. The changes in approach to the care of people with mental handicaps that have occurred during the past two decades have for the most part been driven by ideological concepts, and owe little to detailed consideration of the problems faced by individual handicapped people and their families. The ideas presented by the members of successive committees of enquiry have had a significant impact on current policies, and the need for a vision of the future of services is recognized. The fact that planning and development took place in what was essentially an information vacuum is not necessarily a criticism of those who produced the ideas for change. It was and it remains a major shortcoming of a system in which information has low priority. In this particular field the difficulties are compounded by the large number of organizations and individuals who have some responsibility for people with mental handicaps.

Appendix A

Kensington and Chelsea and Westminster planning register for people with mental handicaps

The registration form is reproduced below in order to illustrate its basic content and structure. It has been reduced in scale and re-typeset but the text remains unchanged.

Service providers need to know basic information about people with mental handicaps to ensure that appropriate services are available when and where people need them. We would be grateful if you could complete this part of the form for anyone who is currently using, or is likely in the future to need to use, services for people with mental handicaps. We aim to update the information every 6 months; so this record is not a static one.

Please write in the spaces in the right hand column, putting only one letter or figure in each space.

<u>CONFIDENTIAL</u>

PART 1 – REGISTRATION

RECORD NO.

1. May this confidential information
   be made available to professionals
   involved in caring or planning
   for this person on request?

   Yes = 1 No = 2

Appendix A

2. **SURNAME**   . . . .

   FIRST NAME: . . . .

   INITIALS of any other forenames   . . . .

3. **SEX:** Male = 1 Female = 2   . .

4. **MARITAL STATUS:**

Single	= 1	Divorced	= 5
Married	= 2	Under age	= 6
Widowed	= 3	Not known	= 7
Separated	= 4	Other	= 8

   . .

   If 'other' (8) please write below:

   ....

5. **DATE OF BIRTH:**   . . | . | . . . .

   Day Month Year

   (e.g. for 2nd June 1940 code)

   .0.2 | 0.6 | 1.9.4.0.
   Day Month Year

6. **LEGAL STATUS:** This person is:

   – under no legal constraint = 01
   – in care = 02
   – under a supervision order = 03
   – on probation = 04
   – the responsibility of a guardian = 05
   – the responsibility of the official solicitor = 06
   – detained under the Mental Health Act = 07
   – none of the above but (please
     specify below) = 08

   . . .

   ....

   – of unknown status = 99

   If coded 07 please state section

   ....

156

7. **RESIDENCE:** This person lives in:

- his/her family home   = 01
- hospital   = 02
- local authority home/hostel for children   = 03
- local authority home/hostel for adults   = 04
- private/voluntary home/hostel for children   = 05
- private/voluntary home/hostel for adults   = 06
- foster home   = 07
- residential school (family home, holidays)   = 08
- independently   = 09
- group home   = 10
- N.H.S. hostel   = 11
- some other place   = 12

Please give details.

....

Is this placement appropriate in your opinion?

Yes = 1 No = 2

8. **ADDRESS:**
   Please give the address of the
   residence referred to in
   question 7.

POSTAL CODE:

If the person with a mental handicap lives with own family or in a foster home (codes 01 or 07 in question 7) please answer question 9. If not, please go to question 10. If independent (09) please go to question 11.

9. **CARER(S) TITLE(S), NAME(S) and AGE:**

Give the title(s), initials (if known), and name(s) of person(s) giving care in the family or foster/adoptive home. If possible we would like the age of the carer(s) recorded too. This gives us one indication of how soon residential provision might be needed.

CARER 1 TITLE and INITIAL(S): | . . . .

NAME: | . . . .

Date of birth of individual
giving care | . . .|.|. . . .
| or estimated age . . .

CARER 2 TITLE and INITIAL(S): | . . . .

NAME: | . . . .

Date of birth of individual
giving care | . . .|.|. .
| or estimated age. . .

PLEASE GO TO QUESTION 11

10. **ADDRESS ON ADMISSION:**
If this person does not live with own family, give family address at the time of <u>first</u> admission to long term institutional care.

. . . .

Date of current admission: | . . . .

Hospital number: | . . . .

Name of ward this person is on: | . . . .

11. **SOCIAL WORK AREA**
Which Social Work Area is responsible for services to this person?
Please write in below.

. . . .

RELIGION

Does this person, or this persons family, belong to any particular religious group?
Please write in below.

....

CULTURAL FACTORS

Are there any strong cultural or religious factors that should be considered when planning for this person?

- – Yes definitely   = 01
- – Yes possibly   = 02
- – Needn't be considered = 03
- – Not known   = 00   . . .

If you need to give more information about these factors, there is space at the end of this form.

12. NEXT OF KIN:

Give title(s), initials, and name of the next of kin of this person with a mental handicap.

               TITLE(S): . . . .

               INITIALS: . . . .

               NAME: . . . .

Please write the relationship of next of kin to the person with a mental handicap (e.g. mother, parents, aunt, brother). If none or not known write below 'none' or 'not known'

....

13. **ADDRESS OF NEXT OF KIN:**

Please write in address of next of kin given in question 12.

If this address has already been
given as the answer to question
8, please tick this box and do
not bother to write in again. ☐
POSTAL CODE:

. . . .
. . . .
. . . .
. . . .
. . . .

14. **GENERAL PRACTITIONER:**

Does the person with a mental handicap have a general practitioner?

Yes = 1 No = 2 Not known = 3   . .

If 'Yes' please give:

SURNAME of general practitioner: . . . .

Address of practice: . . . .

. . . .

. . . .

POSTAL CODE: . . . .

If this person with a mental handicap is in hospital, please answer question 15. If NOT, please go to question 16.

15. **DAY ACTIVITY IN HOSPITAL**: This person is currently:

– attending school = 01
– attending a skills development unit = 02
– attending an industrial workshop = 03
– working on a farm unit = 04
– working on a garden unit = 05
– receiving occupational therapy = 06
      . . .
      Main activity
– receiving behaviour modification
               therapy = 07
– working within hospital = 08
      . . .
– working in open employment = 09
      Other activity

Please write below what type of
employment

....

– in some activity not mentioned above = 10
Please state.

....

– not involved in any activity = 00
– this information is not known = 99
Date of first attendance at main activity   . . |.|. . . .

GO TO QUESTION 18 IN PART 2

16. **SUPPORT & OCCUPATION IF NOT IN HOSPITAL.**

Is the **Community Mental Handicap Team** involved?

Westminster Team = 1
Kensington & Chelsea Team = 2
Out borough Team = 3
None involved = 4
Not Known = 0
  . .

Appendix A

What **financial allowances** is this person receiving?
Please code as below.

Yes = 1   No = 2   Not known = 0

- Supplementary Benefit   `. .`
- Attendance Allowance   `. .`
- Mobility Allowance   `. .`
- Severe Disablement Allowance   `. .`
- Invalid Care Allowance   `. .`
- Other   `. .`

What **daytime occupation** does this person have?

- attending nursery   = 20
- attending day school   = 21
- at a boarding school   = 22
- receiving home teaching   = 23
- attending college   = 24
- on a work experience course = 25   `. . .`
- attending adult training/day/social   Main activity
    education centre = 26   `. . .`
- in sheltered employment   = 27   Other activity
- in open employment   = 28

Please write in employment ....

- other daytime occupation not mentioned above = 29

Please write in occupation ....

- not involved in any daytime activity = 00
- this information is not known   = 99

Date of first attendance at main activity   `. .|.|. . . .`

Is this placement appropriate in your
    opinion?   Yes = 1 No = 2   `. .`

162

Appendix A

17. ADDRESS OF DAY PLACEMENT
(if any)

. . . .

. . . .

. . . .

. . . .

POSTAL CODE: . . . .

PART 2 – ABILITIES

In the next section we need to try to gain an overall picture
of the abilities of this person. As each person is so individual
in what they can and like doing, please could you describe
briefly below his/her main strengths and abilities and ambi-
tions. We will summarize from your words a brief description
to hold on the computer. You will be able to check that you
are happy with this summary. There is more space at the end
of the form should you need it.

....

....

....

....

....

PART 3 – ASSESSMENT

We also need information about any problems this person has in order to plan realistically for facilities and staffing levels.

18. DEGREE OF MENTAL HANDICAP:

Using mental handicap services
    (implied IQ above 70)   = 0
Mild mental retardation
    (I.C.D. code 317 implied IQ 50–70) = 1
Moderate mental retardation
    (I.C.D. code 318.0 implied IQ 35–49) = 2 · ·
Severe mental retardation
    (I.C.D. code 318.1 implied IQ 20–34) = 3
Profound mental retardation
    (I.C.D. code 318.2 implied IQ under 20) = 4
Unspecified mental retardation
    (I.C.D. code 319)   = 5

INTELLIGENCE QUOTIENT
(I.Q.) or Mental Age (M.A)

Please write in any I.Q. test, giving type of test, year tested and where the full results of this test may be obtained.

....

19. ASSESSMENTS

Has this person had a full assessment completed?
Yes = 1 No = 2   · ·

If yes please write in what type of assessment this was (e.g. HALO etc.), the date it was done and where the full results may be obtained.

....

20. **INDIVIDUAL PROGRAM PLAN**

Does this person have an IPP? Yes = 1 No = 2 | . .
                                              | —

If yes please write in the date it was drawn up and where a copy of it may be obtained.

....

21. **DIAGNOSIS:** Please write in below any diagnosis(es) or syndrome(s) thought to be the <u>cause</u> of, or which describe this person's mental handicap (e.g. Down's Syndrome or Microcephaly).

....

....

Please write in below any diagnosis(es) and/or syndrome(s) that <u>complicate the management</u> of this person's life (e.g. Epilepsy or Schizophrenia). If Epilepsy is diagnosed please state whether there are no current fits, fits are controlled with drugs, fits are partially controlled with drugs, fits are uncontrolled even with drugs or not known.

....

....

....

IF THIS PERSON IS A CHILD UNDER 5 YEARS OF AGE QUESTION 22 A–J SHOULD <u>NOT</u> BE COMPLETED. PLEASE TURN TO THE END OF THE FORM AND COMPLETE PART 4

22. A. **CONTINENCE–NIGHTS**

WETTING Frequently = 1 Occasionally = 2 Never = 3 |. .

SOILING Frequently = 1 Occasionally = 2 Never = 3 |. .

CONTINENCE–DAYS

WETTING Frequently = 1 Occasionally = 2 Never = 3 |. .

SOILING Frequently = 1 Occasionally = 2 Never = 3 |. .

B. **MOBILITY**

CAN THIS PERSON WALK WITHOUT HELP

Not at all = 1 Cannot manage stairs = 2
  Can manage stairs and elsewhere = 3   . .

If you have coded 1 or 2, please answer:

CAN THIS PERSON WALK WITH HELP?

Not at all = 1 Cannot manage stairs = 2
  Can manage stairs and elsewhere = 3   . .

IS THIS PERSON WHEELCHAIR DEPENDENT?

No = 1 Yes but cannot manage it = 2
  Yes and can manage it = 3   . .

C. **SELF HELP**

FEED: Not at all = 1 With help or supervision = 2
  Without help = 3   . .

WASH: Not at all = 1 With help or supervision = 2
  Without help = 3   . .

DRESS: Not at all = 1 With help or supervision = 2
  Without help = 3 |. .

D. **VISION:** Blind or almost = 1 Poor = 2
Appears Normal = 3

Has been tested within the last 2 years:
Yes = 1 No = 2

E. **HEARING:** Deaf or almost = 1 Poor = 2
Appears Normal = 3

Has been tested within the last 2 years:
Yes = 1 No = 2

F. **COMMUNICATION**

USE OF SPEECH:

No communication = 1 Asks for basic needs
(eg food, toilet etc) = 2
Asks for more than basic needs = 3

USE OF GESTURE: (if speech is not present, or
if used to augment speech)

No communication = 1 Indicates basic needs
(eg food etc) = 2
Indicates more than basic needs = 3

IF THIS PERSON DOES COMMUNICATE (Codes 2 and
3 above) ARE THESE COMMUNICATIONS:

– difficult to understand even by close
acquaintances; impossible for strangers = 1

– easily understood by close acquaintances;
difficult for strangers = 2

– clear enough to be understod by anyone = 3

CAN THIS PERSON UNDERSTAND SPEECH
OR GESTURE?

Not at all = 1 Basic needs = 2
More than basic needs = 3

G. **LITERACY:** Can the mentally handicapped person

READ AND
UNDERSTAND: Nothing = 1   A little = 2
Newpapers and books = 3   . .

WRITE: Nothing = 1 A little = 2
Own correspondence = 3   . .

COUNT: Nothing = 1 A little = 2
Understands money = 3   . .

H. **COMMUNITY LIVING SKILLS**

SHOPPING/POST OFFICE:

Nothing = 1 With help = 2 On own = 3
No opportunity given = 4   . .

ATTEND CLUBS/SOCIAL EVENTS:

No = 1 With help = 2 On own = 3
No opportunity given = 4   . .

USE TELEPHONE:

No = 1 With help = 2 On own = 3
No opportunity given = 4   . .

USE PUBLIC TRANSPORT:

No = 1 With help = 2 On own = 3
No opportunity given = 4   . .

ROAD SENSE:

None = 2 With help = 2 On own = 3
No opportunity given = 4   . .

Appendix A

We need to know about a person's behaviour for two main reasons. Firstly, to ensure sensible staffing levels in any residential home planned and in psychology and/or other services. Secondly, because people with mental handicaps often have difficulties in speech or signing communication, their behaviour may reflect their anxiety, loneliness, unhappiness, frustration, etc., and its significance should not be ignored. The behaviours listed are some that parents and staff have told us about. If you need to describe other problems, or would like to emphasize the positive aspects of this person's behaviour, please feel free to use the space at the end of the form to do so.

I. **BEHAVIOUR**: Does this person's behaviour cause management problems? For instance,

– is HITTING out or attacking others:

often a severe problem	= 1
occasionally a severe problem	= 2
often a mild problem	= 3
occasionally a mild problem	= 4
never a problem	= 5

– is DAMAGING clothing or furniture:

often a severe problem	= 1
occasionally a severe problem	= 2
often a mild problem	= 3
occasionally a mild problem	= 4
never a problem	= 5

– is EXCESSIVE activity, pacing, disturbed nights:

often a severe problem	= 1
occasionally a severe problem	= 2
often a mild problem	= 3
occasionally a mild problem	= 4
never a problem	= 5

169

Appendix A

- is ATTENTION SEEKING, in that this person will not leave parents or staff:

often a severe problem	= 1
occasionally a severe problem	= 2
often a mild problem	= 3
occasionally a mild problem	= 4
never a problem	= 5

‗‗

- is SELF INJURY (e.g. headbanging, picking at sores etc)

often a severe problem	= 1
occasionally a severe problem	= 2
often a mild problem	= 3
occasionally a mild problem	= 4
never a problem	= 5

‗‗

- are 'DELINQUENT' ACTS (e.g. pilfering, fire, risk, indecent exposure):

often a severe problem	= 1
occasionally a severe problem	= 2
often a mild problem	= 3
occasionally a mild problem	= 4
never a problem	= 5

‗‗

- are PERSONAL HABITS (e.g. masturbation in public, spitting, etc)

often a severe problem	= 1
occasionally a severe problem	= 2
often a mild problem	= 3
occasionally a mild problem	= 4
never a problem	= 5

‗‗

- is WANDERING OFF:

often a severe problem	= 1
occasionally a severe problem	= 2
often a mild problem	= 3
occasionally a mild problem	= 4
never a problem	= 5

‗‗

- is NOISE (e.g. screaming, shouting, verbal aggression, etc):

often a severe problem	= 1
occasionally a severe problem	= 2
often a mild problem	= 3
occasionally a mild problem	= 4
never a problem	= 5

- is the person NEGATIVE, WITHDRAWN or UNCOOPERATIVE to the extent that it is:

often a severe problem	= 1
occasionally a severe problem	= 2
often a mild problem	= 3
occasionally a mild problem	= 4
never a problem	= 5

J. LEVEL OF SUPPORT REQUIRED:

Full time supervision	= 1
Some supervision day and night	= 2
Some supervision during day	= 3
Some supervision during night	= 4
Independent with minimum support	= 5
Independent	= 6

Appendix A

PART 4 – CONTACT

Thank you for the time and trouble you have taken to complete this form. Please could you tell us who you are and where we can contact you, as the register is kept up-to-date by sending a printout of the information currently held to our contact person (or their successor in post) at intervals for checking.

NAME (In capitals please): ....

TITLE/POSITION: ....

PLACE OF WORK/HOME: ....

....

....

....

POSTAL CODE: ....

TELEPHONE NUMBER: ....

Please put the date the form was completed ..|.|....

Please return the completed form to:
  The Register Organisers
  Mrs Jenifer Rohde/Miss Ann Nursey
  Mental Handicap Register
  Department of Community Medicine
  Westminster Medical School
  17 Horseferry Road
  London SW1P 2AR

  Telephone: 071 828 1519

Please use the space below if necessary to give us further information about the person described in this form.

Notes to help you complete the form

The form has been designed to collect the necessary information as accurately as possible with (we hope) the minimum of inconvenience to the person completing it. It looks long but this is because, where possible, explanations are next to the question they refer to.

We return a 'printout' of the information we hold, so that you can check the information is correct. The information is also updated by returning the 'printout' at regular intervals to you or your successor in post for checking. Changes may be made at this or any other time by contacting the register staff.

It is **your** assessment we are interested in, backed up by formal tests if they have been done.

Please write as legibly as possible.

If the person being registered is a child under 5 years of age the questions 22A–J are inappropriate so please do not complete this section of the form.

Guidance on completing the assessment section

If the person is incapacitated due to a temporary injury please code his or her usual ability.

A. CONTINENCE 'Frequently' = More than once a week. Wetting and soiling occurring during an epileptic fit should be recorded in the same way as any other incontinence.

B. MOBILITY This question aims to assess whether a person can walk and how well. If help is needed with walking because he or she is blind or because of danger from fits this should **not** be recorded as an inability to walk.

C. SELF HELP In these questions please code the person as able to do the task 'without help' if undue disturbance is not caused, nor too long taken if the person is left to him or herself.

D. VISION If this person wears spectacles, please assess his or her vision when wearing them.

E. HEARING If this person uses a hearing aid, please assess his or her hearing whilst using it.

G. LITERACY

Reading
– Code 'nothing' if this person is unable to read or recognize his or her own name.
– Code 'a little' if this person can read or recognize his or her own name.
– Code 'newspapers & books' if this person is able to read and understand newspapers or simple books, for instance to find out when a television programme is on. A person who only looks at pictures should be coded as 'nothing'.

Writing
– Code 'nothing' if this person cannot write his or her own name or can only copy it.
– Code 'a little' if this person can at least write their own name without copying it.
– Code 'own correspondence' if he or she can write brief letters or something similar without undue help in composition or the actual process of writing.

Counting
– Code 'nothing' if this person is unable to count or if he or she can count but cannot make any use of it.
– Code 'a little' if this person can recognize small values, for example could lay 5 spoons or fetch 4 sheets.
– Code 'understands money' if he or she can make small purchases at a shop and give or receive correct change.

I. BEHAVIOUR Please code behaviour irrespective of whether the person is prescribed drugs at the time of rating.

'Often' if this behaviour has occurred during the last month and continues to present problems of management.

'Occasionally' if the behaviour occurs between 'often' and 'never'.

'Never' if this behaviour never occurs or so seldom that it is difficult to remember when it last occurred.

'Severe' when this behaviour causes major management problems.

'Mild' if, when this behaviour occurs, it is a nuisance or slight annoyance.

Thank you for completing this form. If you are uncertain about any part of it or need help please telephone Jenifer Rohde or her assistant on 071 828 1519.

References

Adams, M. (1971) *Mental Retardation and its Social Dimensions*, Columbia University Press.

Alaszewski, A. (1988) From Villains to Victims, in *Mental Handicap in the Community* (ed. A. Leighton), Woodhead-Faulkner.

Andersen, E., Fledelius, H.C., Fons, M. *et al.* (1990) An epidemiological study of disability in four year old children from a birth cohort in Frederiksborg County, Denmark. *Dan. Med. Bull.*, **37**(2), 182–5.

Ayers, G.M. (1971) *England's First State Hospitals 1867–1930*, Wellcome Institute.

Baird, P.A. and Sadovnick, A.D. (1985) Mental retardation in over half-a-million consecutive livebirths: an epidemiological study. *Am. J. Ment. Defic.*, **89**(4), 323–30.

Bank-Mikkelson, N.E. (1969) A metropolitan area in Denmark, Copenhagen, in *Changing Patterns in Residential Services for the Mentally Retarded* (eds. R.B. Kugel and W. Wolfensberger), President's Committee on Mental Retardation, Washington DC.

Benassi, G., Guarino, M., Cammarata, S. *et al.* (1990) An epidemiological study on severe mental retardation among school children in Bologna, Italy. *Developmental Medicine for Children*, **32**(10), 895–901.

Bromley Health Authority (1989) *An Enquiry into the circumstances surrounding an accident to a patient with a complex behaviour disorder and a mental handicap.*

Buckley, S. and Sacks, B. (1987) *The Adolescent with Down's syndrome*, Portsmouth Polytechnic.

Cattermole, M., Jahoda, A. and Markova, I. (1988) Leaving home: The experience of People with a Mental Handicap, *Journal of Mental Deficiency Research*, **32**(Part 1), 47–57.

Corbett, J.A. (1979) Psychiatric Morbidity and Mental Retardation, in *Psychiatric Illness and Mental Handicap* (eds. F.E. James and R.P. Snaith), Gaskell.

Cubbon, J.E. and Malin N.A. (1985) *A national survey of Registers of Mentally Handicapped People*, Sheffield City Polytechnic.

Czeizel, A., Sankaranarayanan, K. and Szondy, M. (1990) The load of genetic and partially genetic disease in man. Mental Retardation *Mutation Research*, **232** (2), 291–303.

Delgardo Rodriguez, M., Moreno de la Casa, A., Arenas, M. *et al.* (1989) Prevalence of mental subnormality recorded in the province of Jaen. *Gac. Sanit.*, **3** (10), 327–32.

Diaz-Fernandez, F. (1988) Descriptive epidemiology of registered mentally retarded persons in Galicia (NW Spain). *Am. J. Ment. Retard.*, **92**(4), 385–92.

Dupont, A. (1980) A study concerning the time-related and other burdens when severely handicapped children are reared at home. *Acta Psych. Scand.*, **62**, 249–57.

Elliott, D., Jackson, D.M. and Graves, J.P. (1981) The Oxfordshire Mental Handicap Register. *BMJ*, **282** (6266), 789–92.

Elwood, J.H. and Darragh, B.M. (1981) Severe mental handicap in Northern Ireland. *Journal of Mental Deficiency Research*, **25**, (Part 3) 147–55.

Eyman (1990) Life Expectancy of Profoundly Handicapped People with Mental Retardation. *New England Journal of Medicine*, pp. 584–9.

Farmer, R.D.T. and Rohde, J.R. (1983) A register of mentally handicapped individuals using a microcomputer. *Journal of Mental Deficiency Research*, **27**, 255–78.

Farmer, R.D.T., Holroyd, S. and Rohde, J.R. (1990) Differences in disability between people with mental handicaps who were resettled in the community and those who remain in hospital. *BMJ*, **301**, 646.

Fleming, I. and Stenfert Kroese, B. (1990) Evaluation of a community care project for people with learning disabilities. *Journal of Mental Deficiency Research*, **34**, (Part 6) 451–64.

Fryers, T. (1984) *The Epidemiology of Severe Intellectual*

impairment, Academic Press.

Fryers, T. (1987) Epidemiological issues in mental retardation. *Journal of Mental Deficiency Research*, **31**, (Part 4) 365–84.

Fryers, T. (1990) Mental Retardation and Epidemiology. *Current Opinion in Psychiatry*, **3** (5), 595–602.

Gostason, R. (1985) Psychiatric illness among the mentally retarded. A Swedish population study. *Acta Psychiatr. Scand. Suppl.*, **318**, 1–117.

Gustavson, K.H., Holmgren, G., Jonsell, R. *et al*, (1977). Severe mental retardation in children in a Northern Swedish County. *Journal of Mental Deficiency Research*, **21**, 161–80.

Hagberg, B. and Kyllerman, M. (1983) Epidemiology of mental retardation – a Swedish survey. *Brain Development*, **5**, 441–9.

Hagberg, G., Lewerth, A., Olsson, E. *et al*. (1987) Mild mental retardation in Gothenburg children born between 1966–1970. Changes between two points of time, *Ups. J. Med. Sci. Suppl.*, **44**, 52–7.

Herbst, D.S. and Baird, P.A. (1983) Nonspecific mental retardation in British Columbia as ascertained through a registry. *Am. J. Ment. Defic.*, **87**, 506–13.

HMSO (1959) Mental Health Act.

HMSO (1971) *Better Services for the Mentally Handicapped, Cmnd 4683*, DHSS and Welsh Office, London.

HMSO (1979) *The Jay Report – Report of the Committee of Enquiry into Mental Handicap Nursing and Care.*

HMSO (1989) *Caring for People – Community Care in the next Decade and Beyond, Cm 849.*

Ineichen, B. (1984) Prevalance of Mental Illness amongst Mentally Handicapped People, *JRSM*, **77**, 761–5.

Jahoda, M., Cattermole, M. and Markova, I. (1990) Moving out: an opportunity for friendship and broadening social horizons? *Journal of Mental Deficiency Research*, **34**, 127–39.

Joyce, C., Marsh, R.W. and Thompson, G.B. (1988) The prevalence of mental handicap in New Zealand. *NZ Medical Journal*, **101**, 660–2.

Kanner, L. (1943) Autistic disturbances of affective contact. *Nerv. Child.*, **2**, 217–50.

Kushlick, A. and Cox, G.R. (1973) The epidemiology of mental handicap. *Developmental Medicine and Child Neurology*, **15**, 748–59.

References

Kushlick, A., Blunden, R. and Cox, G.A. (1973) A method of rating behaviour characteristics for use in large scale surveys of mental handicap. *Pyschological Medicine*, **3**, 466.

Locker, D., Rao, B. and Weddell, J.M. (1984) Evaluating community care for the mentally handicapped adult: a comparison of hostel, home and hospital care. *Journal of Mental Deficiency Research*, **28**, 189–98.

Mallon, J.R., MacKay, D.N., McDonald, G. *et al.* (1991) The prevalence of severe handicap in Northern Ireland. *Journal of Mental Deficiency*, **35**, 66–72.

Martindale, A. (1976) A Case Register as an Information System in a Development Project for the Mentally Handicapped. *British Journal of Mental Subnormality*, **22**, 70–6.

Martindale, A. (1980) The distribution of the mentally handicapped between districts of a large city. *British Journal of Mental Subnormality*, **26**, 9–20.

McGrother, C.W. and Marshall, B. (1990) Recent trends in incidence, morbidity and survival in Down's syndrome. *J. Ment. Def. Research.*, **34**, 49–58.

McLoughlin, I.J. (1988) A study of mortality experiences in a mental-handicap hospital. *Br. J. Psychiatry*, **153**, 645–9.

McQueen, P.C., Spence, M.W., Garner J.B. *et al.* (1987) Prevalence of major mental retardation and associated disabilities in the Canadian Maritime Provinces. *American Journal of Mental Deficiency*, **91**, 460–6.

Miller, E. Nicoll, A. Rousseau, S.A. *et al.* (1987) Congenital rubella in babies of South Asian women in England and Wales: an excess and its causes. *BMJ*, **294**, 737–9.

Neligan, G., Prudham, D. and Steiner, H. (1974) *The Formative Years*, Nuffield/OUP, London.

North West Thames Regional Health Authority (1990) *Report of the Inquiry Team into the Resettlement of Long-Stay Psychiatric Patients from St Bernard's Hospital.*

Nursey, A., Rohde, J.R. and Farmer, R.D.T. (1990) Words used to refer to mental handicap: a comparison of parents' and doctors' views. *Mental Handicap*, **18**, 30–32.

O'Brien, K.F., Tate, K. and Zaharia, E.S. (1991) Mortality in a large southeastern facility for persons with mental retardation. *Am. J. Ment. Retard.*, **95**(4), 397–403.

References

Parsons, C.G. (1963) West Indian Babies with multiple congenital defects. *Archives Dis. Childhood*, **38**, 454–8.

Pueschel, S.M. and Mulick, J.A. (eds) (1990) *Prevention of Developmental Disabilities*, Paul Brooks.

Puras, D.K. (1987) Severe mental retardation in an urban child population. *Zh. Nevropatol. Psikhiatr.*, **87**(3), 389–92.

Rantakallio, P. and von Wendt, L. (1986) Mental retardation and subnormality in a birth cohort of 12 000 children in Northern Finland. *Am. J. Ment. Defic.*, **90**, 380–7.

Richards, B.W. and Siddiqui, A.Q. (1980) Age and mortality trends in residents of an institution for the mentally handicapped. *Journal of Mental Deficiency Research*, **24**, 99–105.

Simila, S., von Wendt, L. and Rantakallio, P, (1986) Mortality of mentally retarded children to 17 years of age assessed in a prospective one-year birth cohort. *Journal of Mental Deficiency*, **30**, 401–5.

Williams, C.E. (1971) A study of the patients in a group of mental subnormality hospitals. *British Journal of Mental Subnormality*, **17**, 19–41.

Wing, L. (1972) Services for the mentally retarded, in *Evaluating a Community Psychiatry Service* (eds J.K. Wing and A.M. Hailey), OUP, London.

Wing, L. (1989) *Hospital Closure and the Resettlement of Residents: The Case of Darenth Park*, Gower.

Wolf, L.C. and Wright, R.E. (1987) Changes in life expectancy of mentally retarded persons in Canadian institutions: a 12-year comparison. *Journal of Mental Deficiency Research*, **31**, 41–59.

Wolfensberger, W. (1972) *The Principle of Normalisation in Human Services*, National Institute of Mental Retardation.

Index

Page numbers in italic represent tables, those in bold represent figures

hospital residents 71–2
LA home residents 97
NHS hostel residents 104–5
P/V home residents 86
Immigration 43
Immunization 1, 43
Incidence 14, *27*, 118
Incontinence, *see* Continence
Independent living 33, 107,
112–13
    age distribution *108*
    day activities *109*
    degree of mental handicap
    109
Industrial workshop *63*, *64*
Information systems 14, 138,
151–4
    see also Registers
Inpatients, *see* Hospital
    residents
Institutions 3
Intellectual impairment, *see*
    Degree of mental
    handicap
Intelligence Quotient (IQ) *26*,
141–2
International Classification of
    Diseases, *see* ICD9
Intranatal care 1, 140

Jay Report, The (1979) 6

Kensington Chelsea &
    Westminster Area Health
    Authority (KCWAHA)
    14–15, 138

LA homes 32, 90–9, **125**, *135*,
149
    age at admission 92
    age distribution **91**
    behaviour *96*
    blind 95

communication 95
comparison with all others
    98
continence *94*
day activities *94*
deaf 95
degree of mental handicap
    93
disabilities, combinations of
    97
illustrative cases 97–8
length of stay 92
literacy 95
mobility *95*
self-help skills 95, *96*
sensory function 95
severe behaviour problems
    97
speech 95
Learning disability or
    difficulty, *see*
    Terminology
Life expectancy
    carers 42–3
    Down's syndrome 118
    people with mental
        handicaps **24**
    profound mental handicap
        23
Limitations of estimates of
    prevalence 28
Literacy
    family home residents 48–9
    foster home residents *110*
    group home residents *110*,
        114
    hospital residents 67–8
    independent living *110*
    residents in other
        accommodation *110*
    LA home residents 95
    P/V home residents 84
    residential school pupils *110*

sensory function 84
severe behaviour problems
86
speech 84
wheelchair *83*

Quality 89

Rates
age specific *19*
death 21, *23*
registration 17
Read, *see* Literacy
Readmissions 9
Regional Health Authority, *see*
North West Thames
Registers ix, 12, 14–16, *18, 19,*
138
Registration 17, *18, 19*
Resettlement 58, 63, 99, 100,
146
Residence, place of 31–8
age distribution (%), in *35*
autism **125**
disability, severity of 133–5,
135
districts % use *37*
Down's syndrome **119**
family home 31, 39–56
foster homes 32–3
group homes 34
hospital 31–2, 57–75
independent living 33
LA homes or hostels 32, 90–9
NHS hostels 34, 100–6
numbers in age groups **36**
other types of
accommodation 34,
107–15, 114
P/V homes or hostels 32,
76–89
residential schools 33
Residential schools 33, 44, 107,

111–12
age distribution *108*
day activities *109*
degree of mental handicap
109
Residents in
family homes 39–56, **119**,
135
foster home 107–11, **119**
group home 107
hospitals 57–75, **119**, *135*
independent living 107, **119**
LA homes and hostels 90–9,
119, *135*
NHS hostels *100–6*
other *107–15*, **119**, *135*
P/V homes 76–89, **119**, *135*
residential schools 107
Royal Commission (1908) 3
Royal Commission on law
relating to Mental Illness
and Mental Handicap
(1957) 4
Royal Society for Mentally
Handicapped Children
and Adults, *see* MENCAP
Rubella 43

School, *see* Day school;
Residential school
Scores, disability 51
SECs 12, 44, 82, 94, 150
Segregation 3, 5
Self-help skills
family home residents *49*
foster home residents *110*
group home residents *110*
hospital residents 68–9
independent living *110*
LA home residents 95, *96*
NHS hostel residents 103
other accommodation,
residents in *110*